The EMDR Coloring Book for Kids

The EMDR Coloring Book for Kids
A Resource for Therapists, Parents, and Children

Mark Odland - MA, LMFT, MDIV

Bilateral Innovations
Minnesota

Copyright © 2018 by Mark Odland

All rights reserved. No part of this book may be reproduced, stored in a retrieval system, or transmitted in any form or by any means, electronic, mechanical, photocopying, recording, or otherwise, without the prior permission of Bilateral Innovations.

Published in the United States by Bilateral Innovations
www.bilateralinnovations.com
mark@bilateralinnovations.com

Artwork printed with permission from publicdomainvectors.com

Names: Odland, Mark, author.
Title: The EMDR Coloring Book for Kids: A Resource for Therapists, Parents, and Children
Description: First American edition. Minnesota: Bilateral Innovations, an assumed name of North Woods Christian Counseling, LLC, [2018]
BISAC: Medical / Mental Health

ISBN-13:   978-1719321754
ISBN-10:   1719321752

Content available as a Paperback Book.

PRINTED IN THE UNITED STATES OF AMERICA

10 9 8 7 6 5 4 3 2 1

First American Edition

PREFACE

The Purpose of this Book

The EMDR Coloring Book for Kids provides a fun, creative, and accessible way for children to engage in the EMDR therapy process. Incorporating coloring, drawing, and positive affirmations, it can be used to identify a child's memory targets, strengthen internal resources, and provide emotional grounding both in and outside of therapy sessions.

How to Use This Book

During Phase 1 of the EMDR therapy Standard Protocol (Client History), ask your clients to complete drawings in the "My Resources" and "What Might Need to Heal" sections of the book *(the order in which they complete these drawings will be determined by your clinical judgment based on the unique needs of your clients)*. These completed drawings will give you valuable information about the following:

1) <u>Internal Resources</u> that could later be installed with bilateral stimulation as part of Phase 2 (Preparation)

2) <u>Potential Memory Targets</u> that could later be processed as part of EMDR therapy phases 3-6 (Assessment - Body Scan).

During Phase 7 (Closure), you can instruct your clients to color a page from the "Coloring the Truth" section of the book. By coloring a simple image paired with a positive affirmation, this activity can serve as a grounding or calming resource. You might also instruct them to do this between sessions. However, the book's use as a calming resource would still be seen as a compliment to other established resources like the "Calm/Safe Place" or "Container."

<u>Disclaimer</u>

*Any encouragement for a client to use this book outside of the therapy office is, of course, a matter of your clinical judgment. It will be based on each client's unique history and the support system available to them. For one client, completing the entire "What Might Need to Heal" section could be done at home in the presence of a loving and supportive parent. For another, a variety of factors might make using the book at

home destabilizing. It should also be made clear to parents that the book itself is not EMDR therapy, and that it is no substitute for actual therapy sessions with you.

How the Positive Affirmations were Selected

The positive self-statements in the "Coloring the Truth" section of this book were inspired by the positive "cognitions" listed in EMDR therapy basic trainings. These core affirmations and their variants will be familiar to EMDR therapists around the world because they depict the types of statements clients want to believe as they heal from their trauma. While some of these statements might not technically meet the definition of a "cognition," they've been included because of their potential to be helpful and encouraging.

How the Artwork was Chosen

In contrast to the first two EMDR Coloring Books for adults, for this new book I intentionally selected images that would be more child friendly. The 40 images contained in the "Coloring the Truth" section of this book primarily include images from nature, like animals and flowers (*all taken from publicdomainvectors.com*). To account for children with shorter attention spans, the images are simple and do not take long to color. My hope is that the book will allow children to have fun with the coloring process, while at the same time reinforcing the positive statement written above it. Although the pages are not perforated, the images are purposefully printed only on one side, allowing individual pages to be cut or ripped out. I sincerely hope that this book is an encouragement to therapists, parents, and children around the world, and that it plays some small role in the EMDR therapy healing process.

Blessings,

Mark Odland - MA, LMFT, MDIV

CONTENTS

9 **Section 1: My Resources**

11	A Time I Felt Happy	101	A Time I Felt Ugly
13	A Time I Felt Peaceful	103	A Time I Felt Jealous
15	A Time I Felt Loved	105	A Time I Felt Serious
17	A Time I Felt Excited	107	A Time I Felt Worthless
19	A Time I Felt Curious	109	A Time I Felt Misunderstood
21	A Time I Felt Like a Hero		
23	A Time I Felt Safe	111	**Section 3: Coloring the Truth**
25	A Time I Felt Brave		
27	A Time I Felt Tough	113	I am Worth It
29	A Time I Felt Forgiven	115	I am Special
31	A Time I Felt Hopeful	117	I am Loved
33	A Time I Felt Attractive	119	I am Forgiven
35	A Time I Felt Thankful	121	I am Accepted
37	A Time I Felt Like Laughing	123	I can Learn
39	A Time I Felt Important	125	I am Lovable
41	A Time I Felt Listened To	127	I am Valuable
43	Someone That Makes me Happy	129	I can Make Mistakes
45	Someone That Loves Me	131	I am Fine
47	Someone That is Fun	133	I Made It
49	My Favorite Hero	135	I Matter
51	Someone That is Safe	137	I Have Choices
53	Someone That is Brave	139	I am Stronger Now
55	Someone That is Tough	141	I am a Hero
57	Someone That Forgives Me	143	I am Smart
59	Someone That I'm Thankful For	145	I am Brave
61	Someone That is Funny	147	I am Okay
		149	I am Tough
63	**Section 2: What Might Need to Heal**	151	I Did the Best I Could
		153	I am Strong
65	My Family	155	I am Beautiful
67	My Friends	157	I Can Handle It
69	My Home	159	I Have What it Takes
71	My School	161	I Can Learn
73	Me	163	I Tried
75	If My Wish Came True	165	I am Better Now
77	If I Had One Super Power	167	I Can Change
79	A Time I Felt Sad	169	I Deserve Good Things
81	A Time I Felt Worried	171	I am Strong Now
83	A Time I Felt Unloved	173	I am Worthy
85	A Time I Felt Bored	175	I am Unique
87	A Time I Felt Disgusted	177	I can Face my Fears
89	A Time I Felt Like a Bad Person	179	I am Wonderful
91	A Time Someone Seemed Angry	181	I Can do It
93	A Time I Felt Scared	183	I am Alright
95	A Time I Felt Weak	185	I Believe in Myself
97	A Time I Felt Guilty	187	I Can Grow
99	A Time I Felt Discouraged	189	I Can Become Stronger

MY RESOURCES

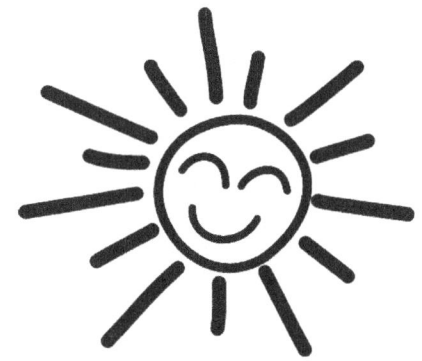

A Time I Felt Happy

A Time I Felt Peaceful

A Time I Felt Loved

A Time I Felt Excited

A Time I Felt Curious

A Time I Felt Like a Hero

A Time I Felt Safe

A Time I Felt Brave

A Time I Felt Tough

A Time I Felt Forgiven

A Time I Felt Hopeful

A Time I Felt Attractive

A Time I Felt Thankful

A Time I Felt Like Laughing

A Time I Felt Important

A Time I Felt Listened To

Someone That Makes me Happy

Someone That Loves Me

Someone That is Fun

My Favorite Hero

Someone That is Safe

Someone That is Brave

Someone That is Tough

Someone That Forgives Me

Someone That I'm Thankful For

Someone That is Funny

WHAT MIGHT NEED TO HEAL

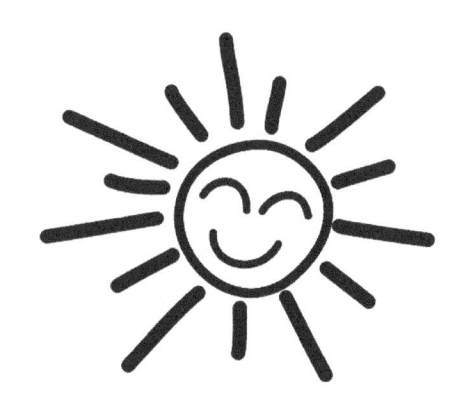

My Family

My Friends

My Home

My School

Me

If My Wish Came True

If I Had One Super Power

A Time I Felt Sad

A Time I Felt Worried

A Time I Felt Unloved

A Time I Felt Bored

A Time I Felt Disgusted

A Time I Felt Like a Bad Person

A Time Someone Seemed Angry

A Time I Felt Scared

A Time I Felt Weak

A Time I Felt Guilty

A Time I Felt Discouraged

A Time I Felt Ugly

A Time I Felt Jealous

A Time I Felt Serious

A Time I Felt Worthless

A Time I Felt Misunderstood

COLORING THE TRUTH

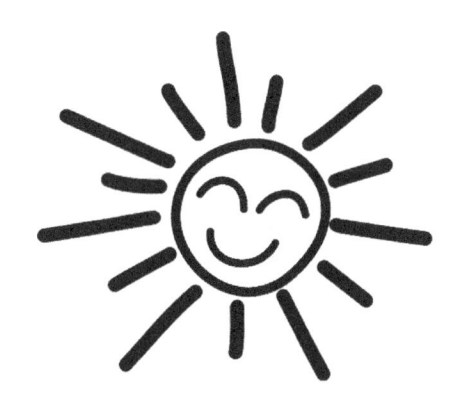

I am Worth It

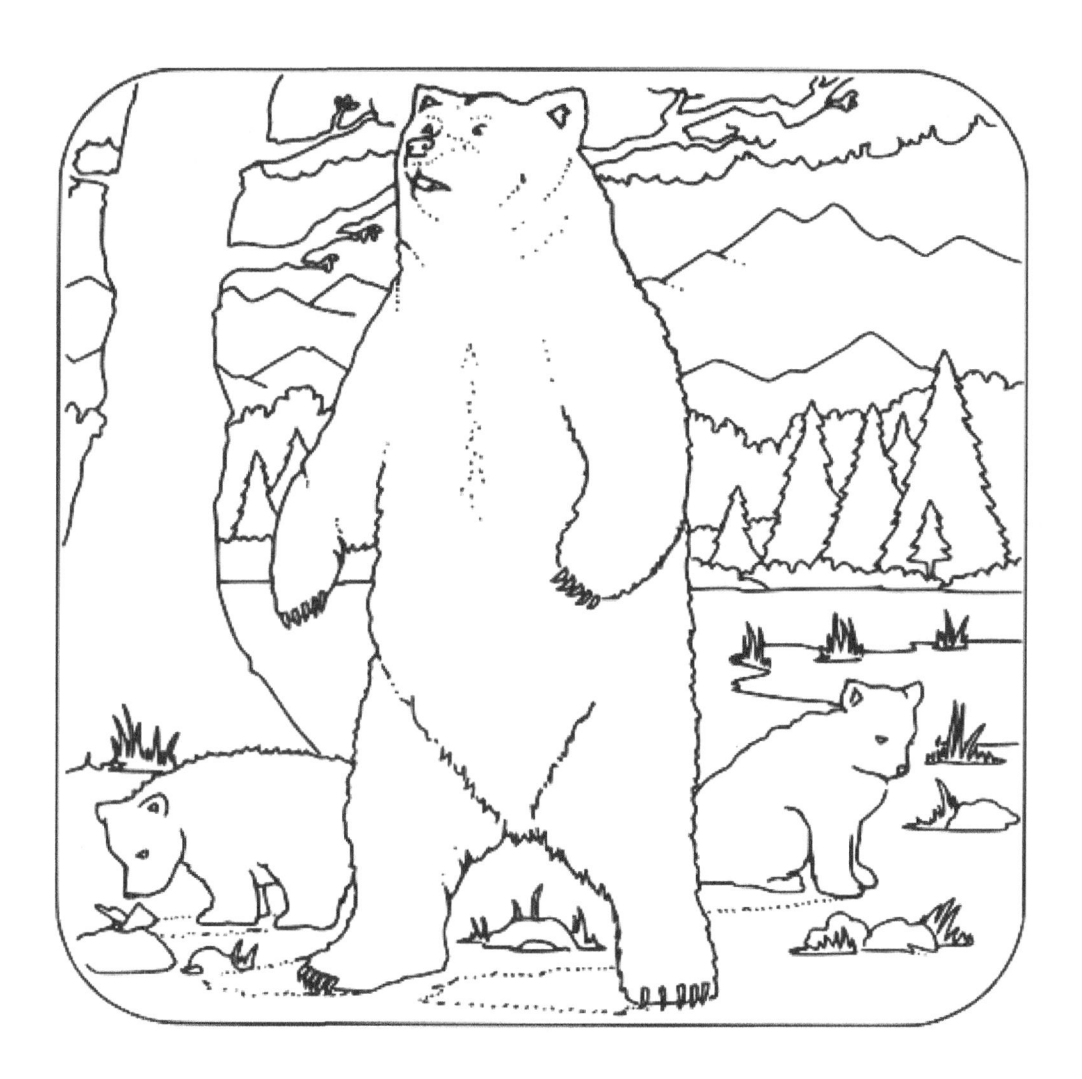

I am Special

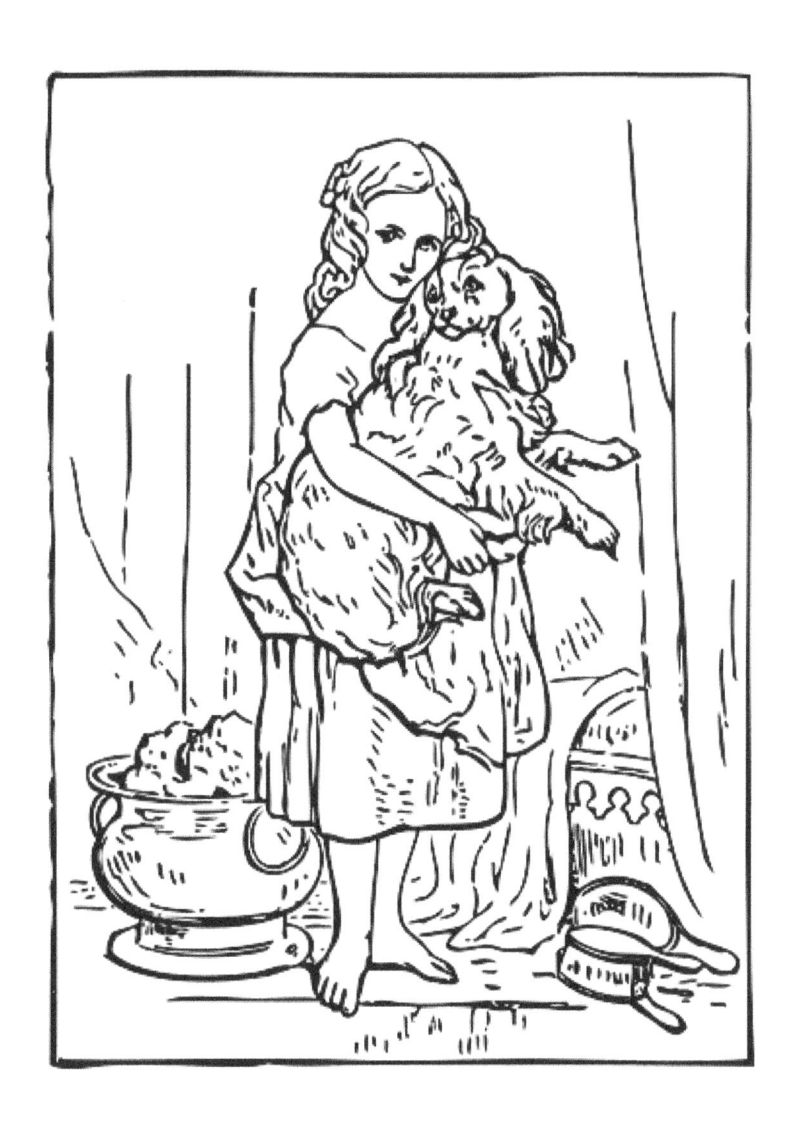

I am Loved

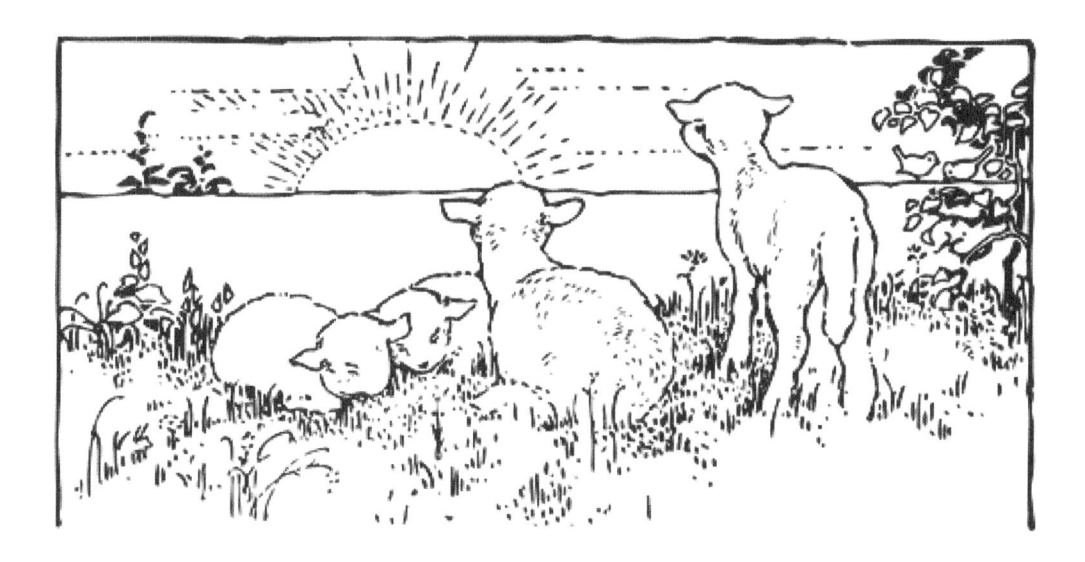

I am Forgiven

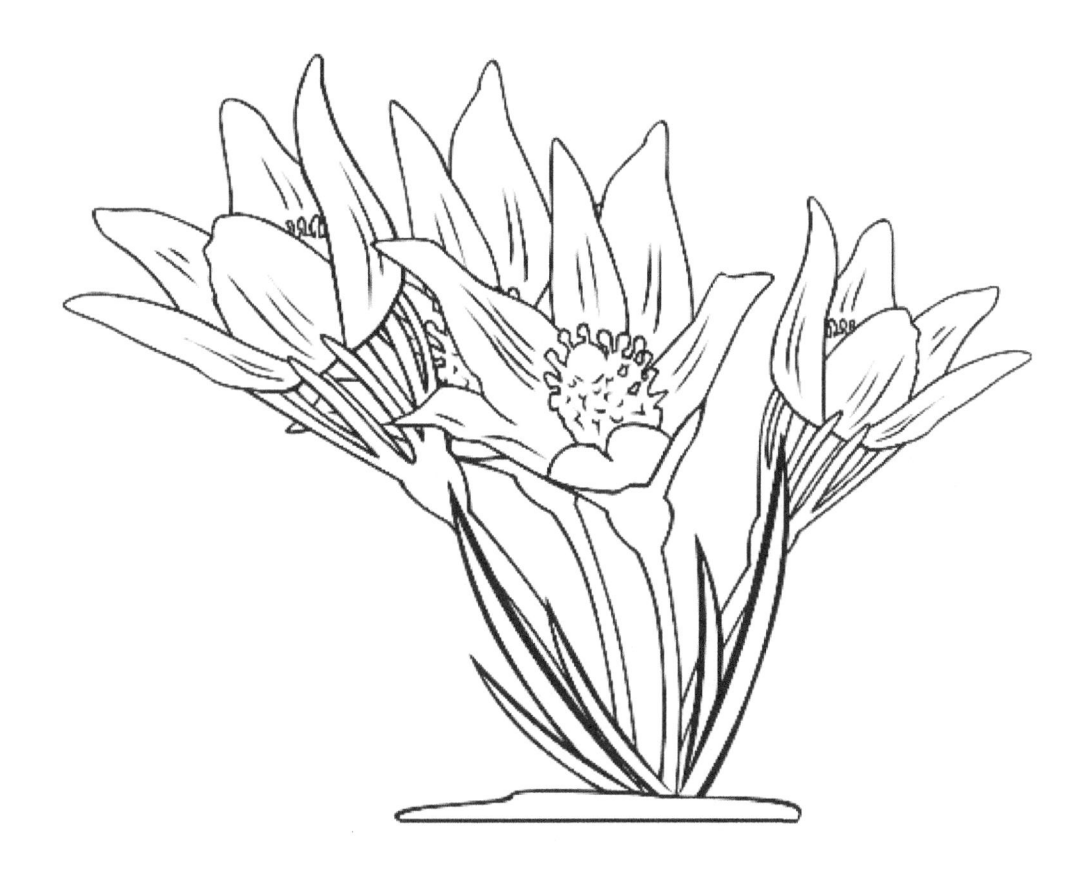

I am Accepted

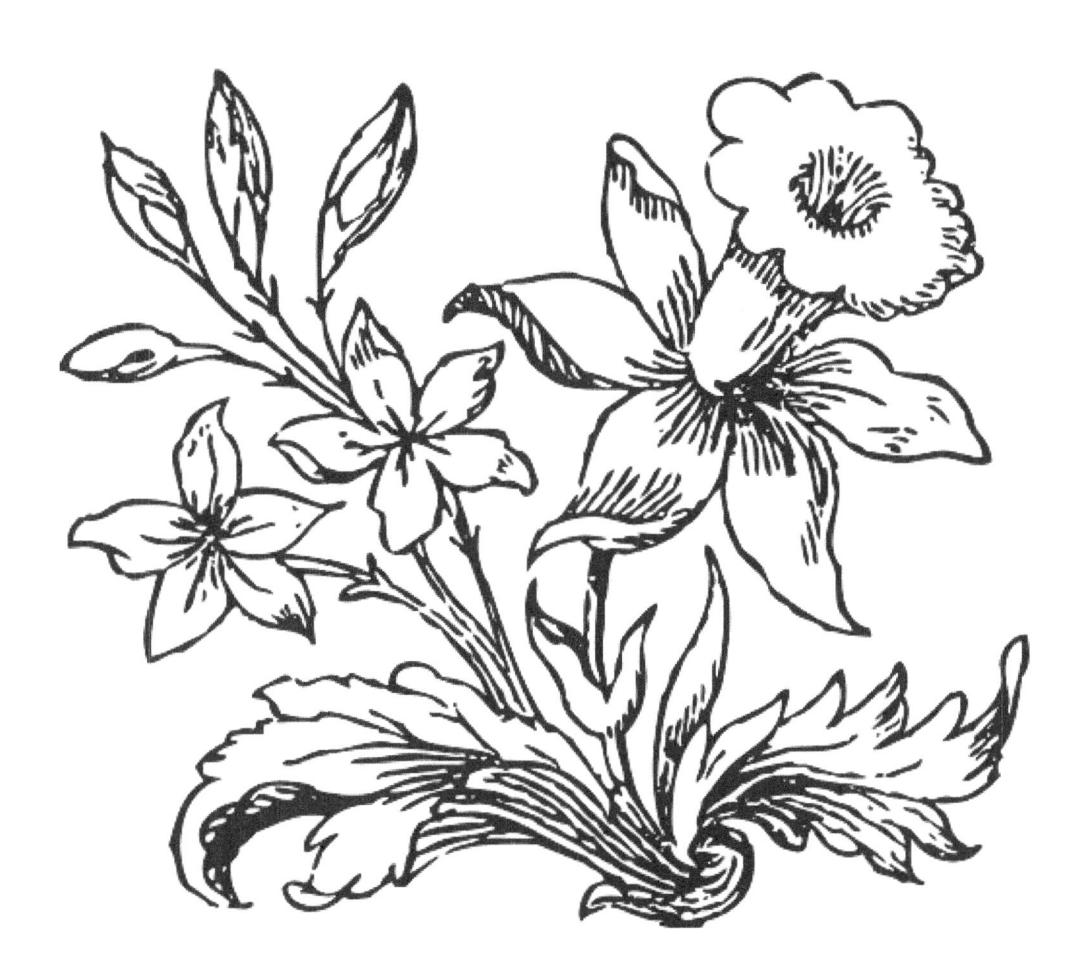

I can Learn

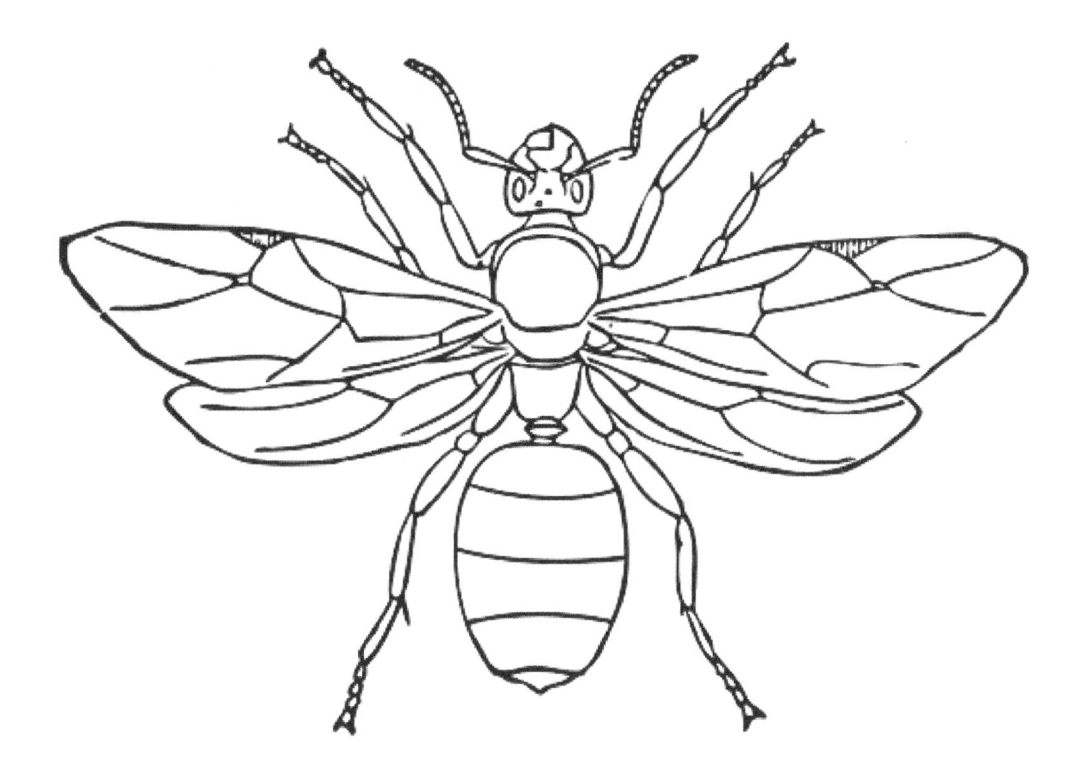

I am Lovable

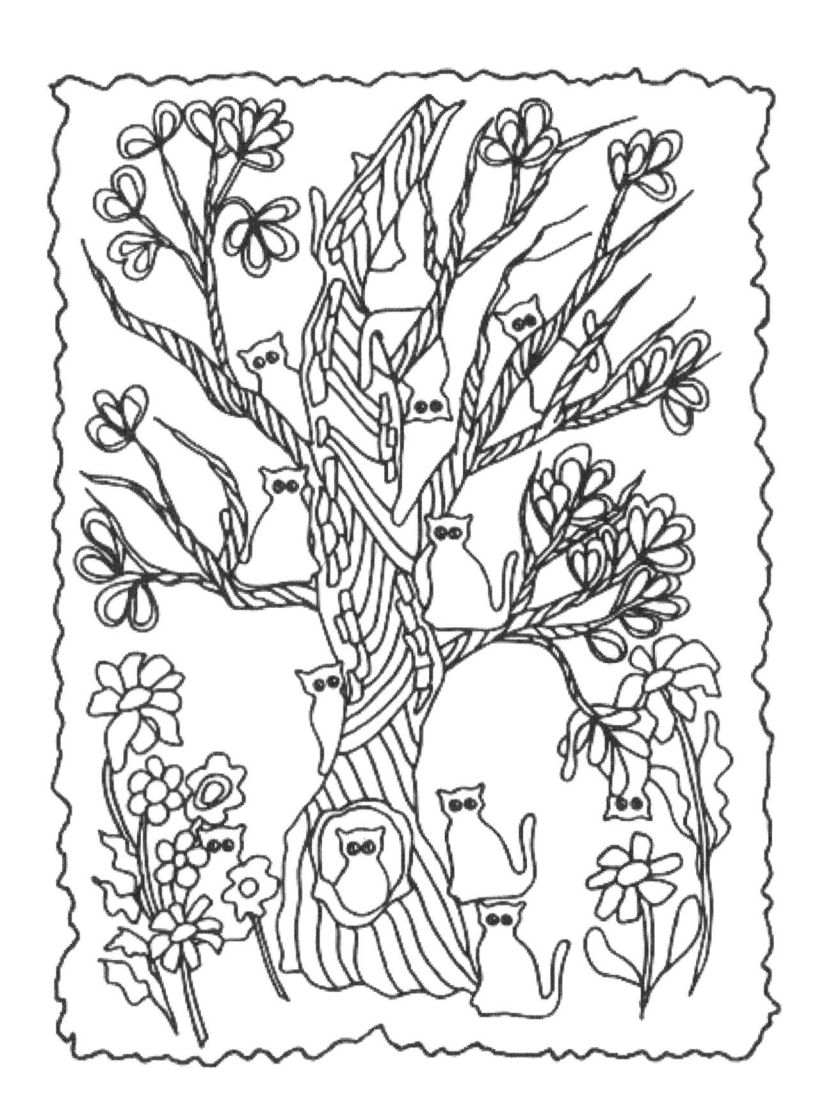

I am Valuable

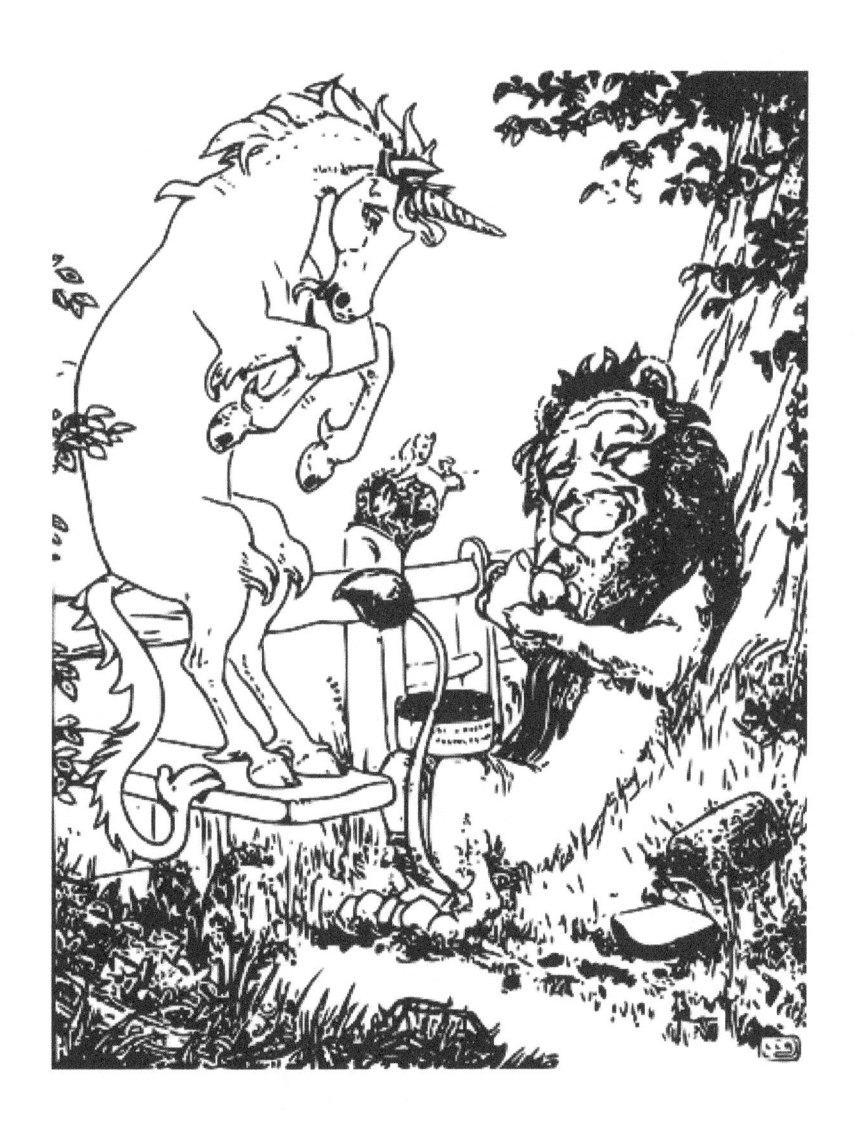

I can Make Mistakes

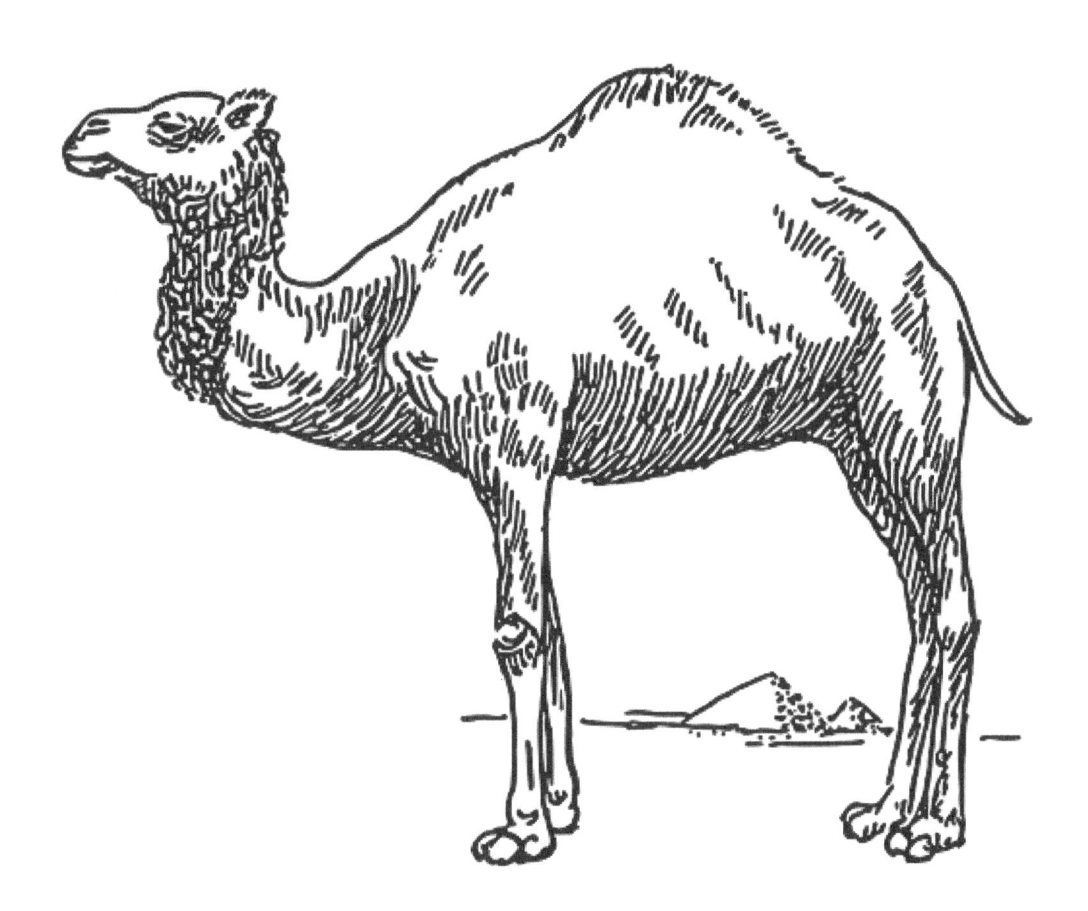

I am Fine

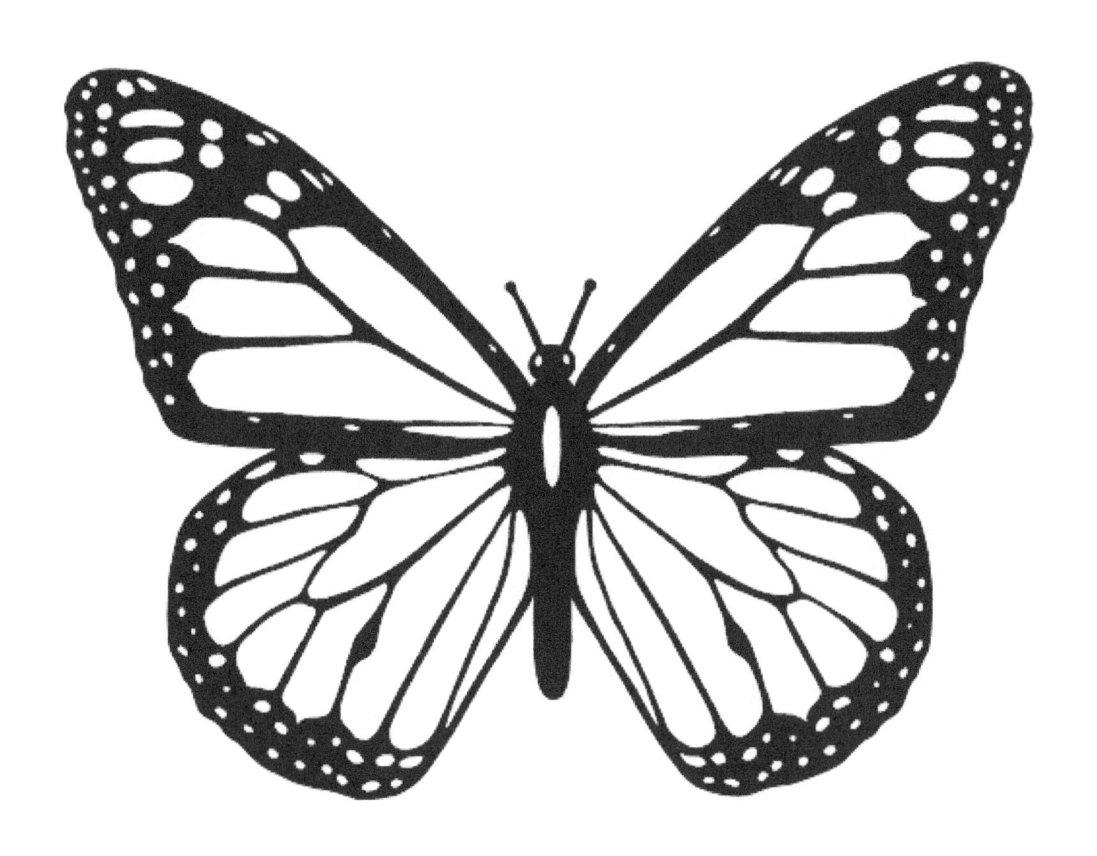

I Made It

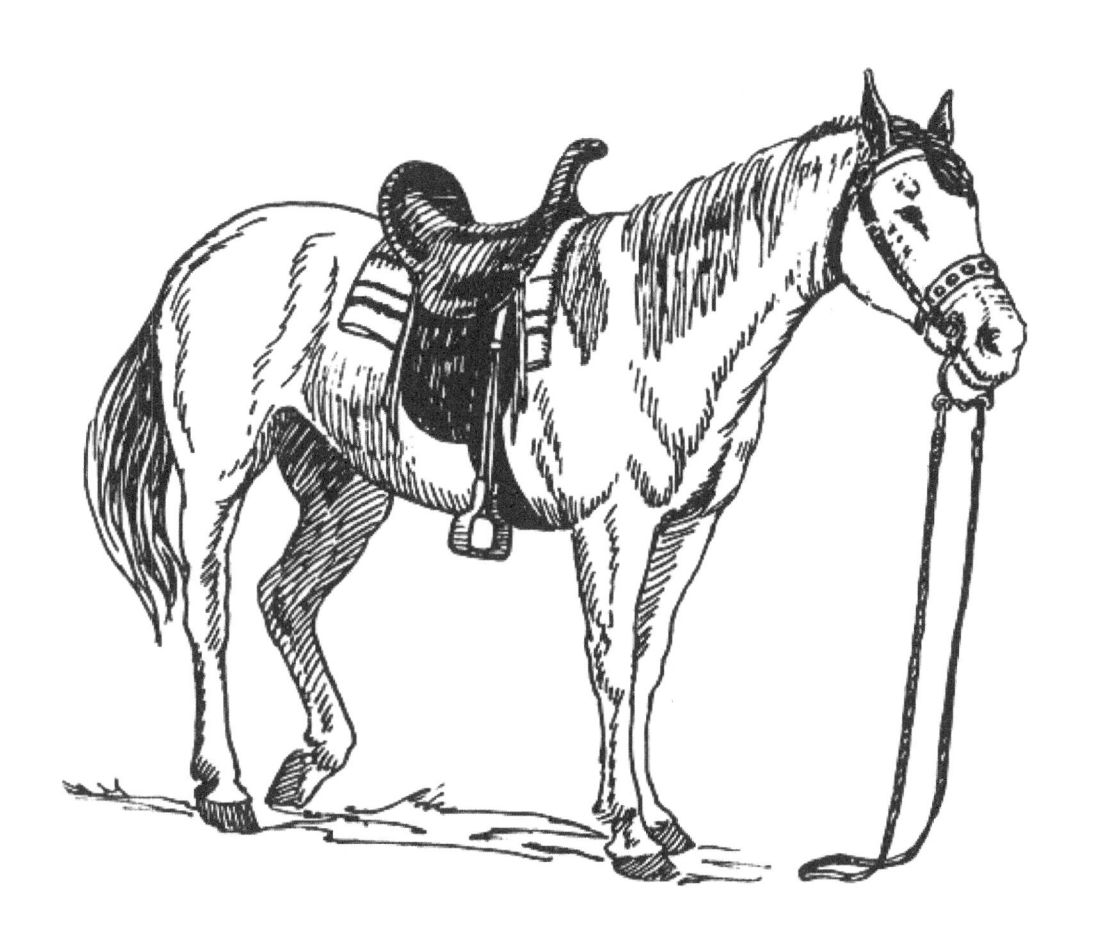

I Matter

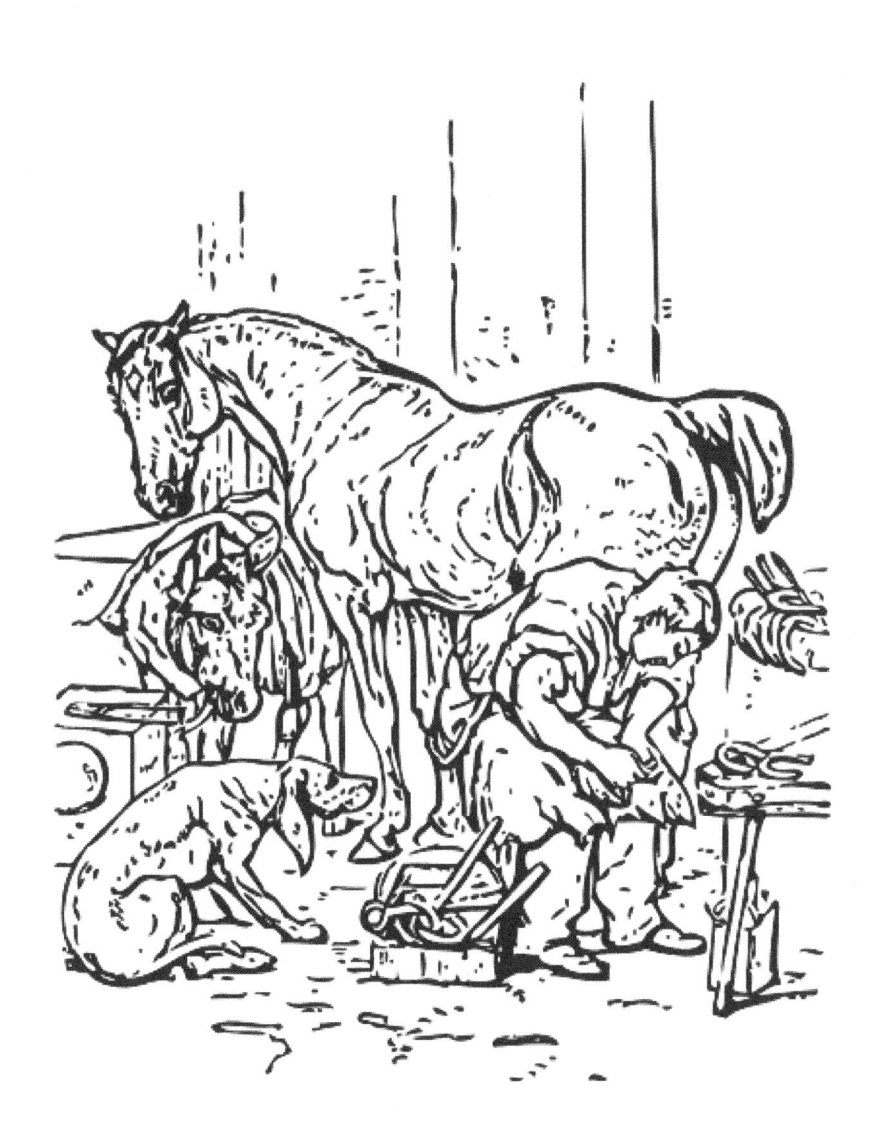

I Have Choices

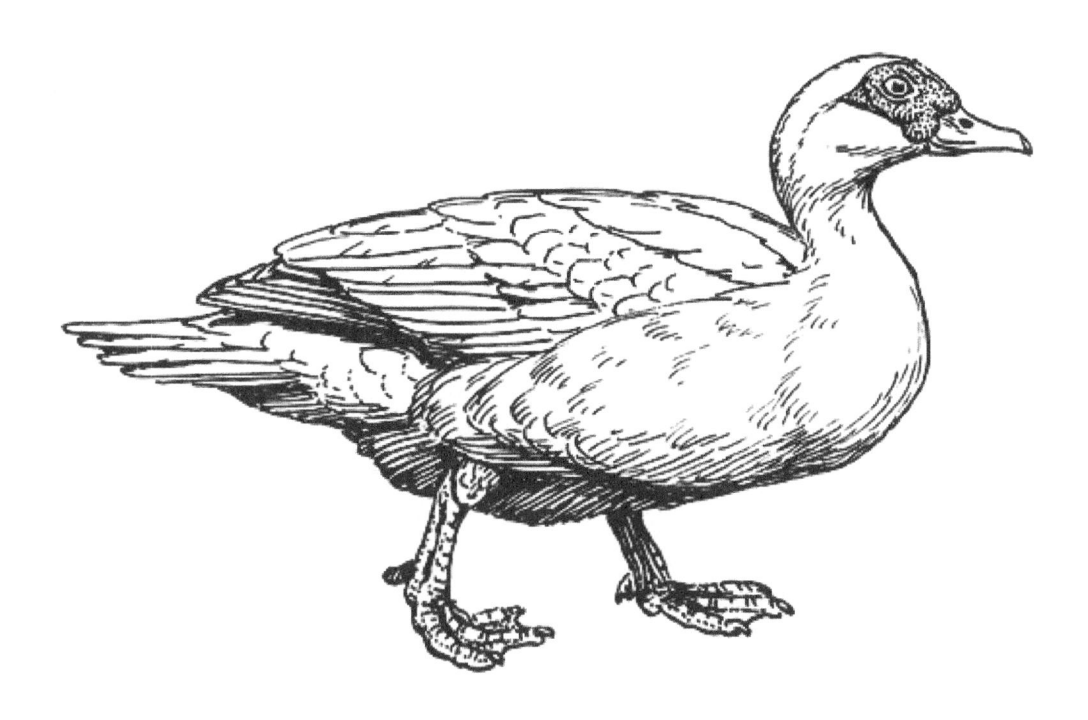

I am Stronger Now

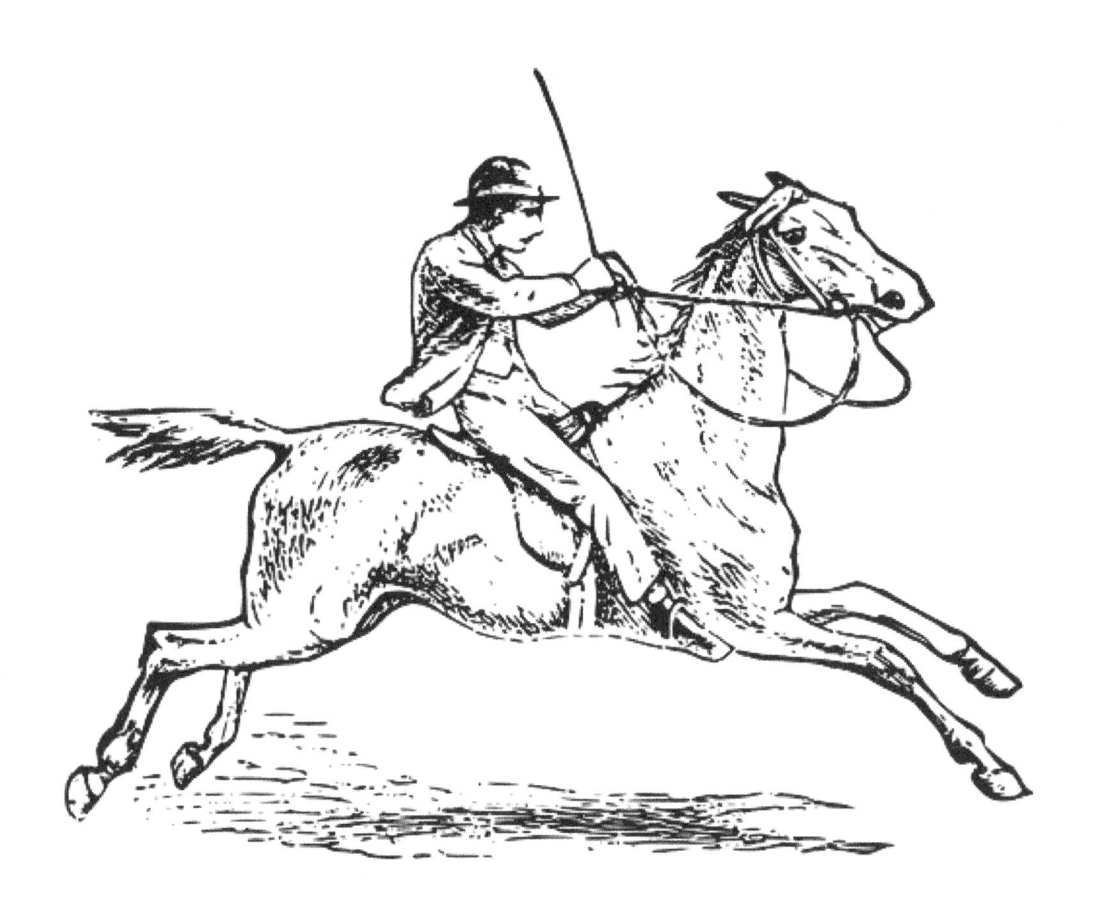

I am a Hero

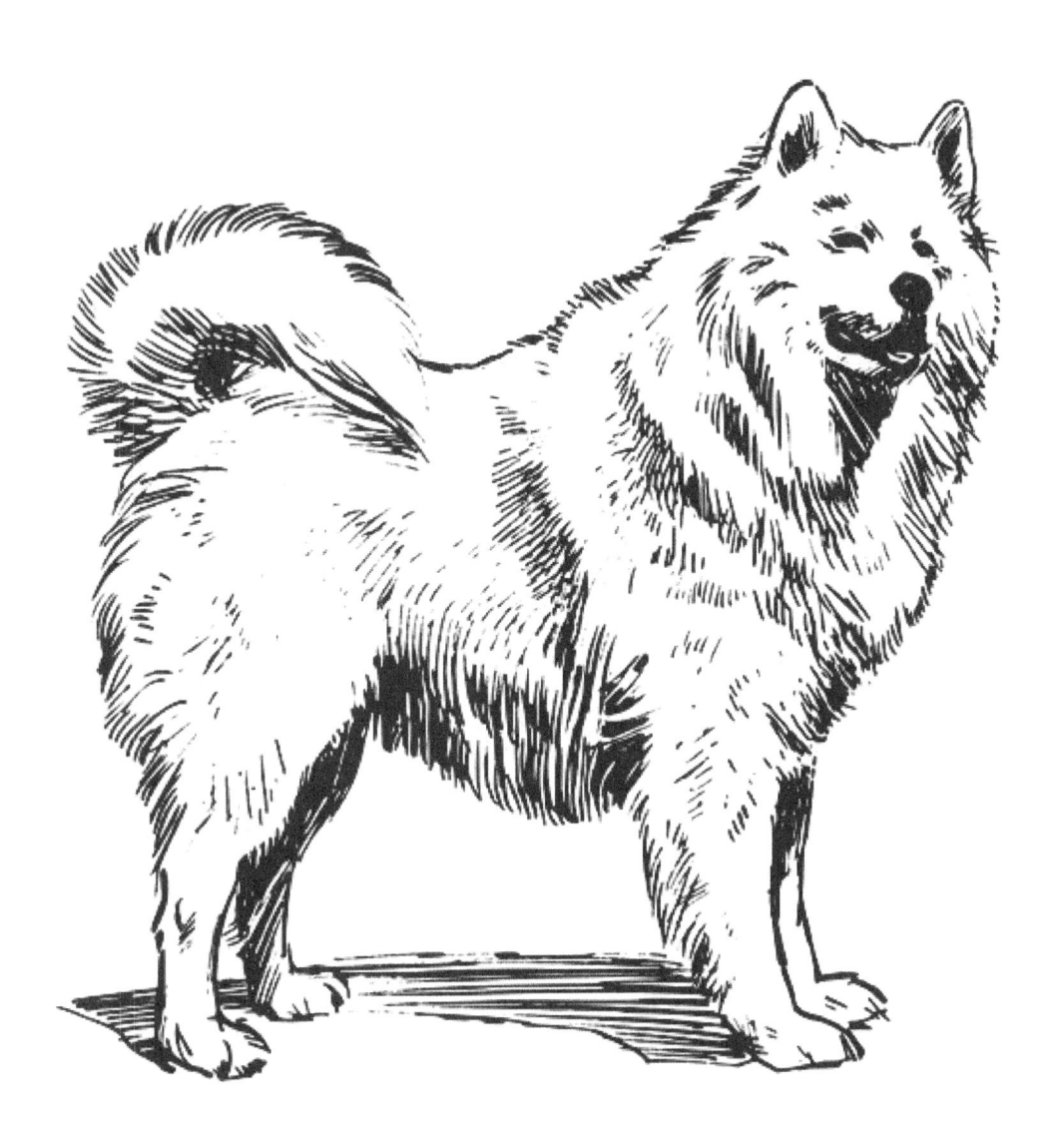

I am Smart

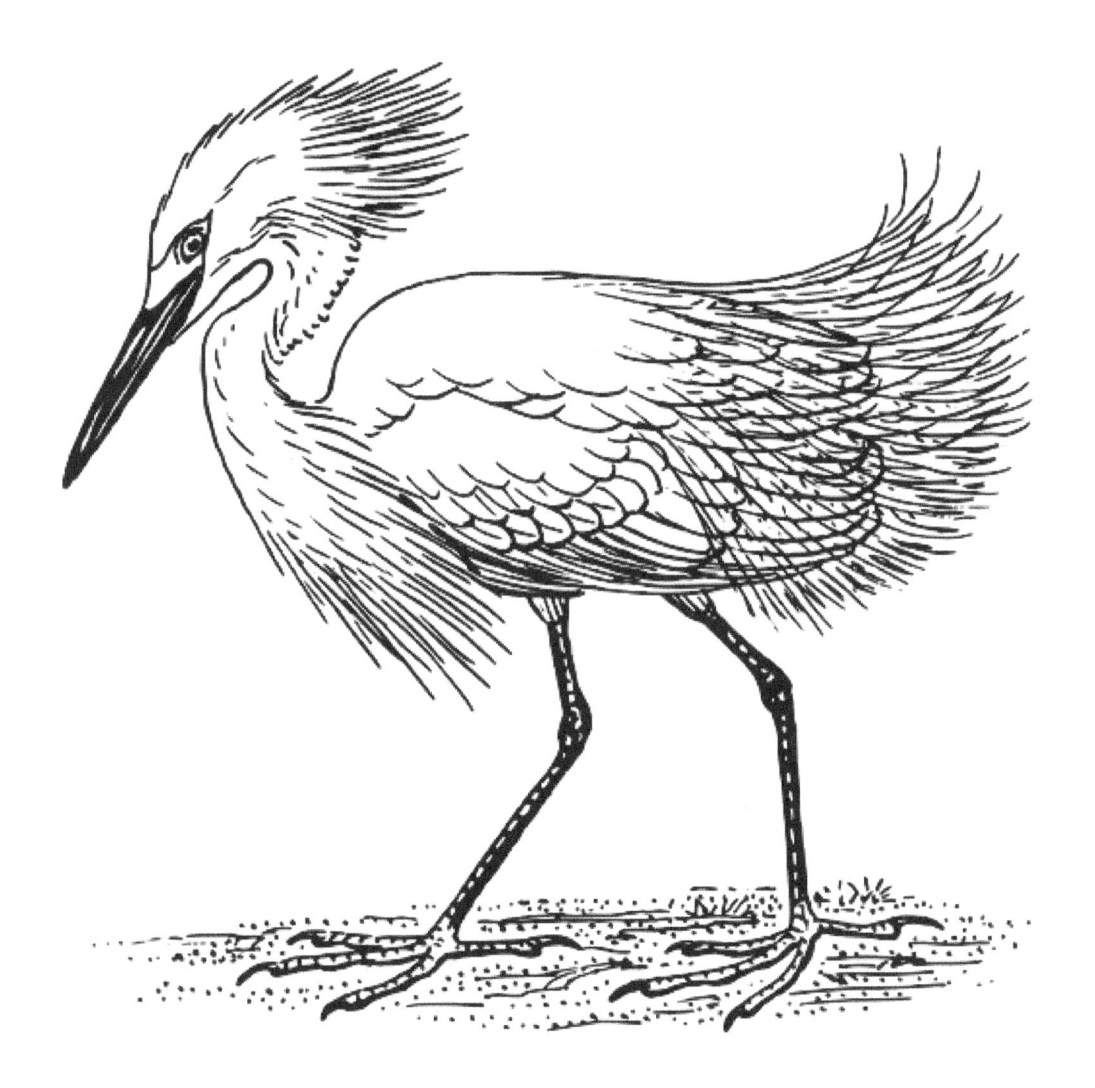

I am Brave

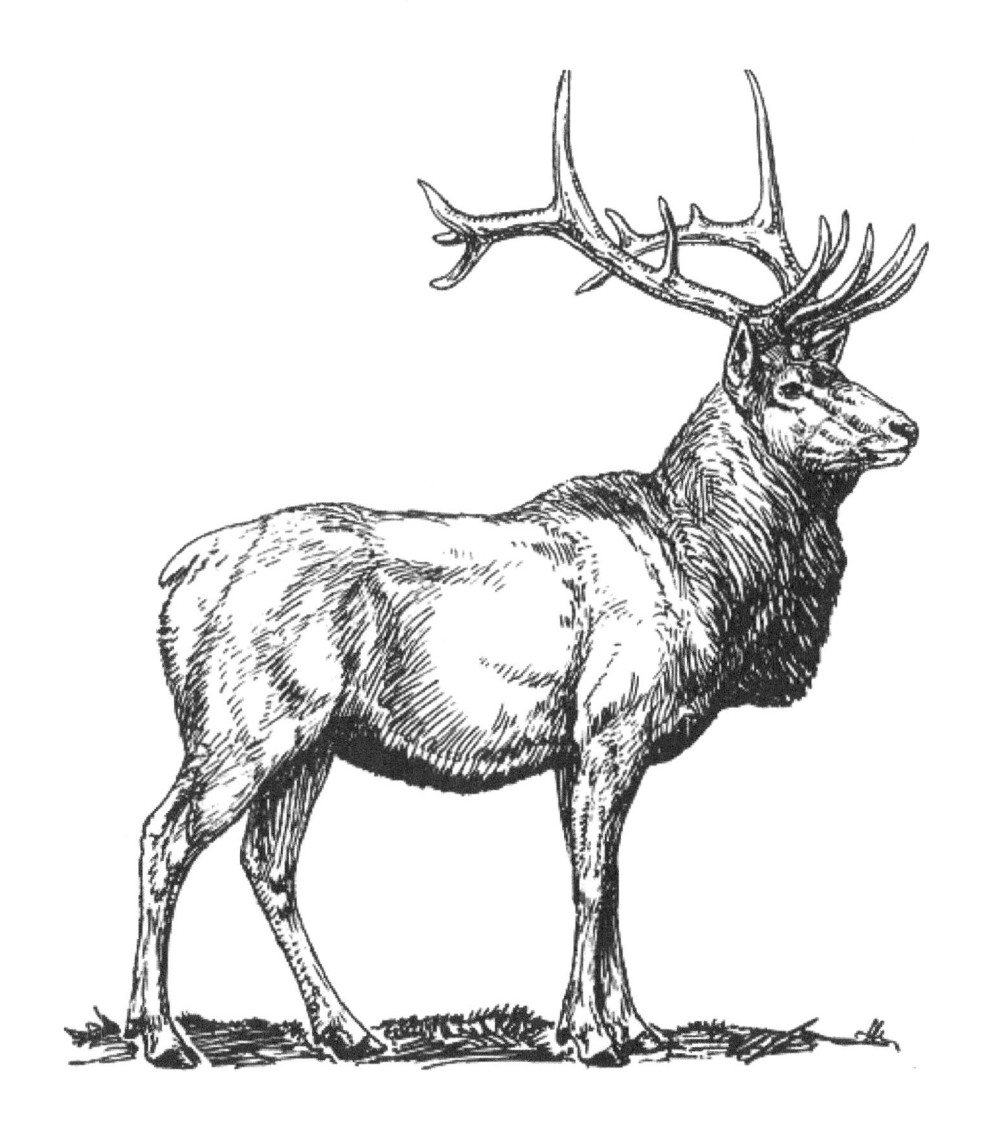

I am Okay

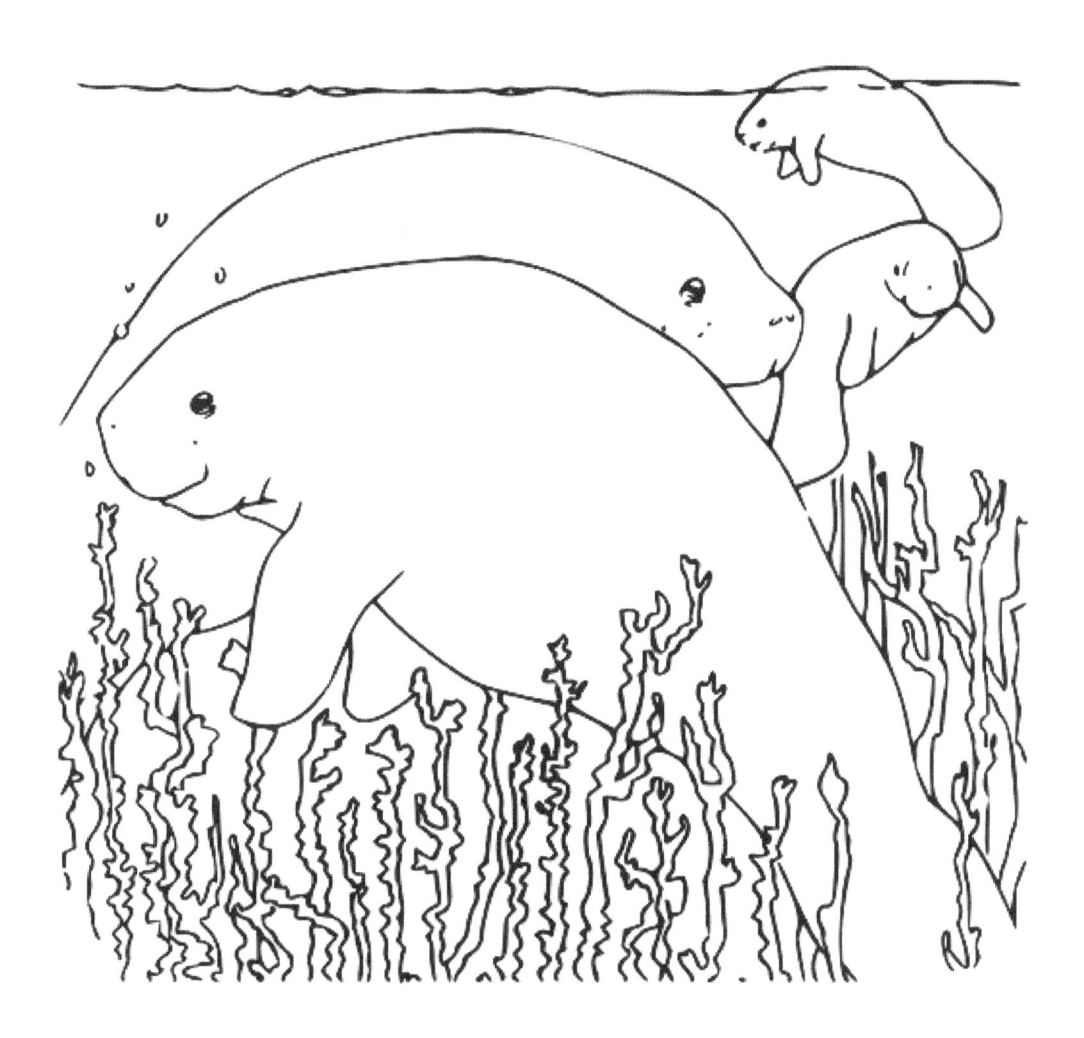

I am Tough

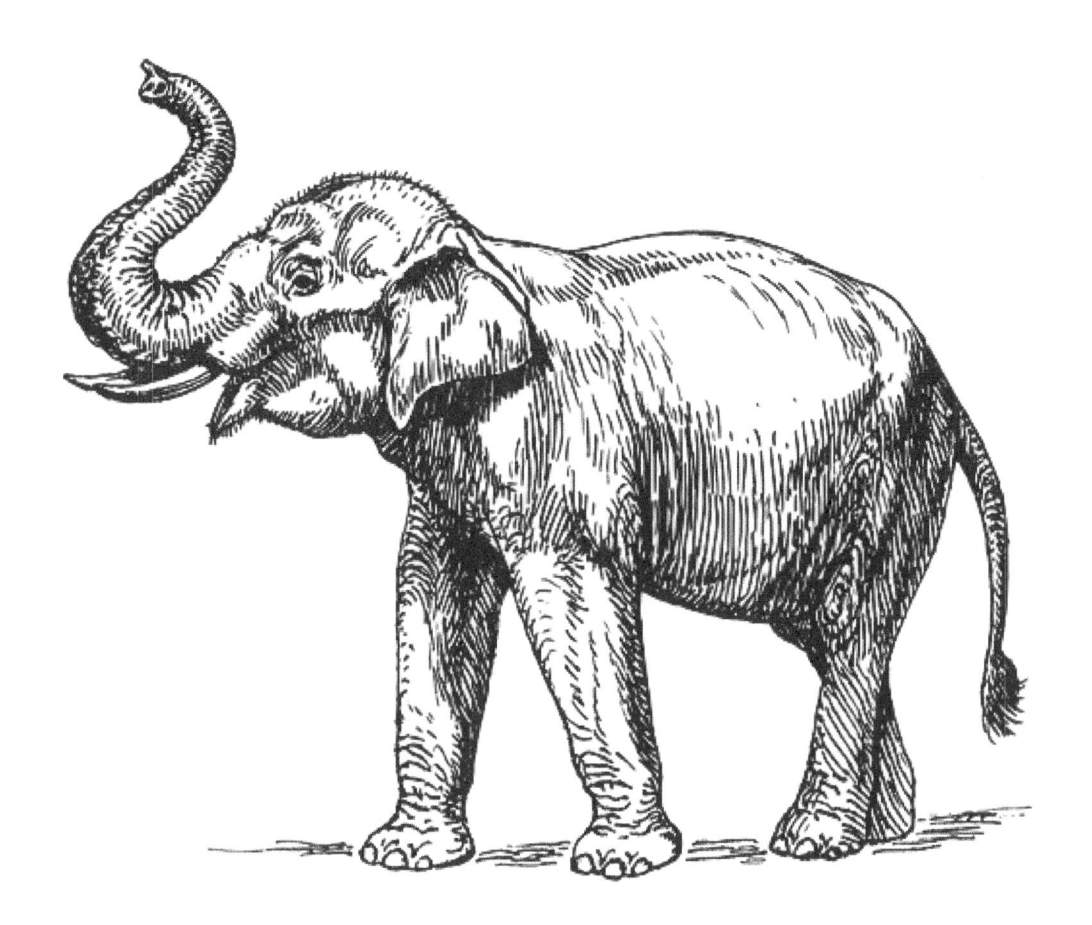

I Did the Best I Could

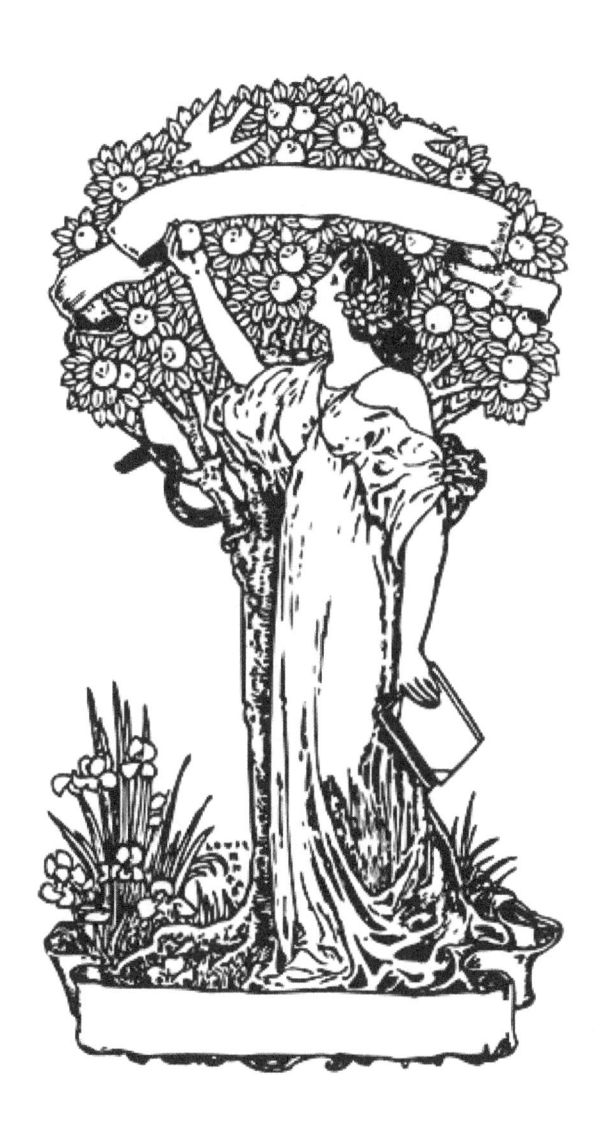

I am Strong

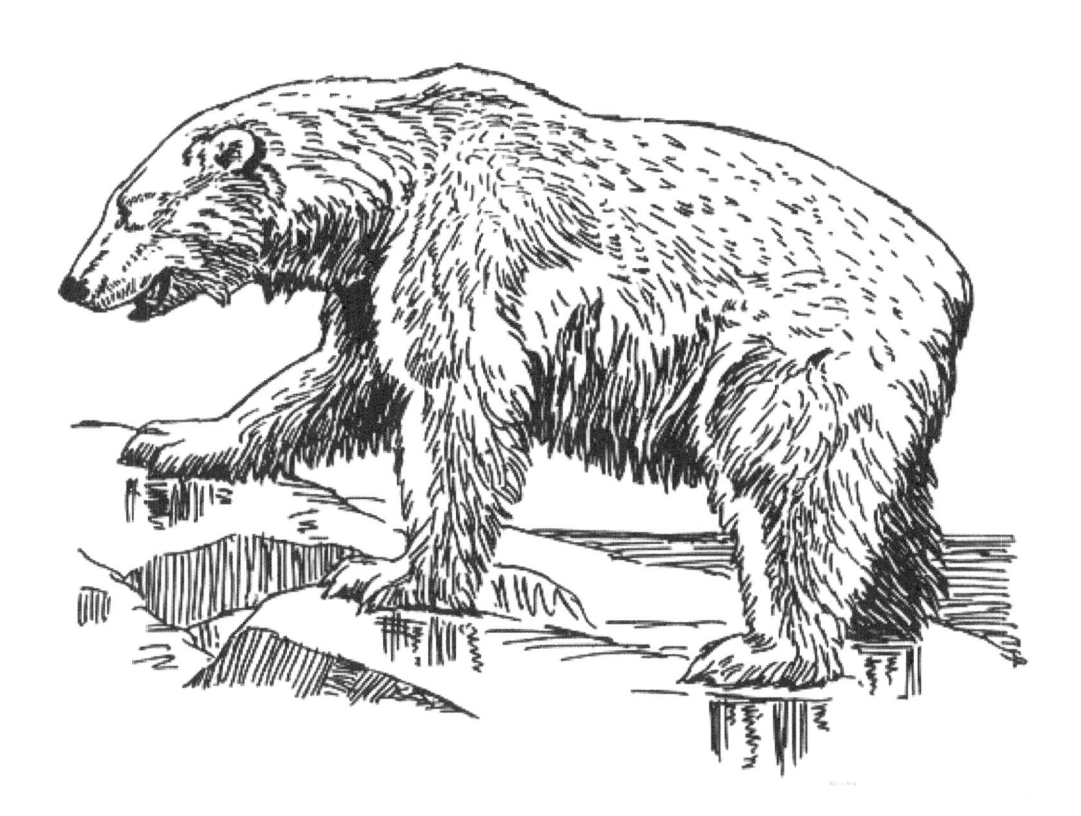

I am Beautiful

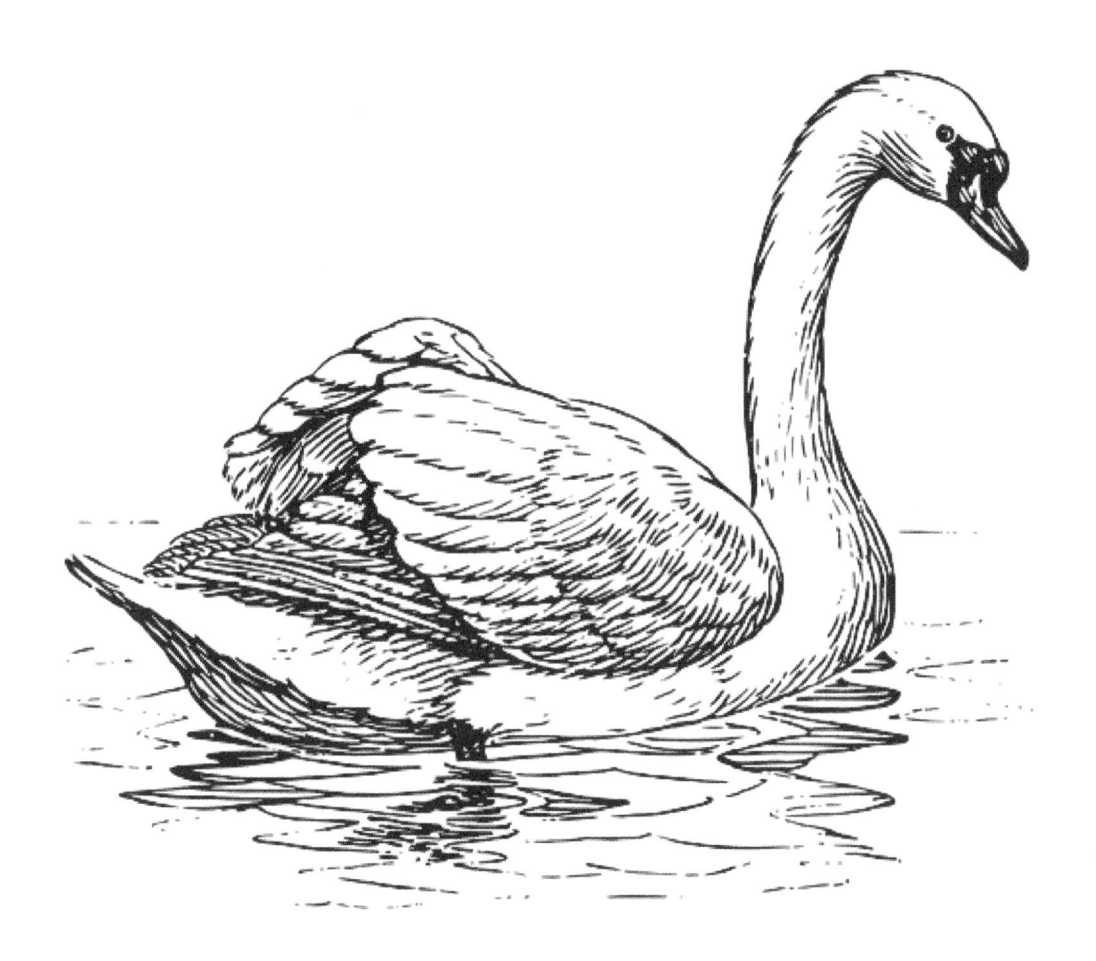

I Can Handle It

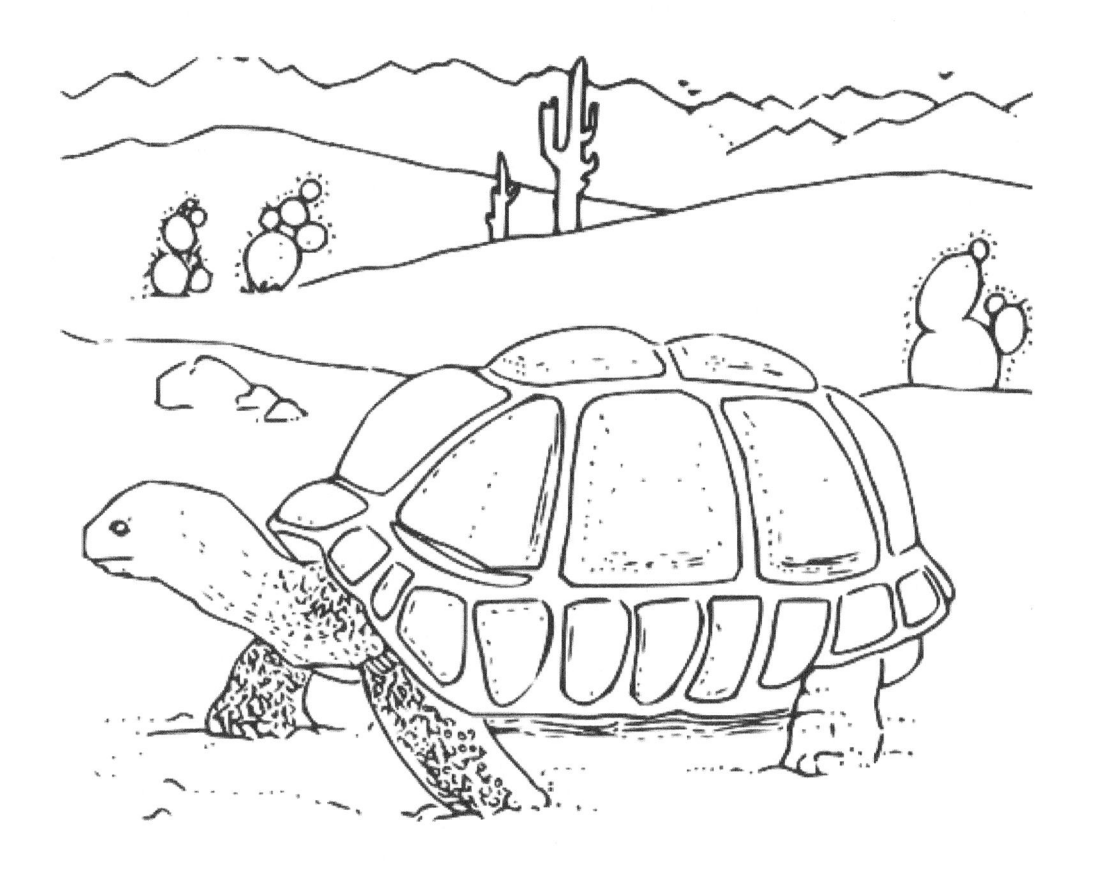

I Have What it Takes

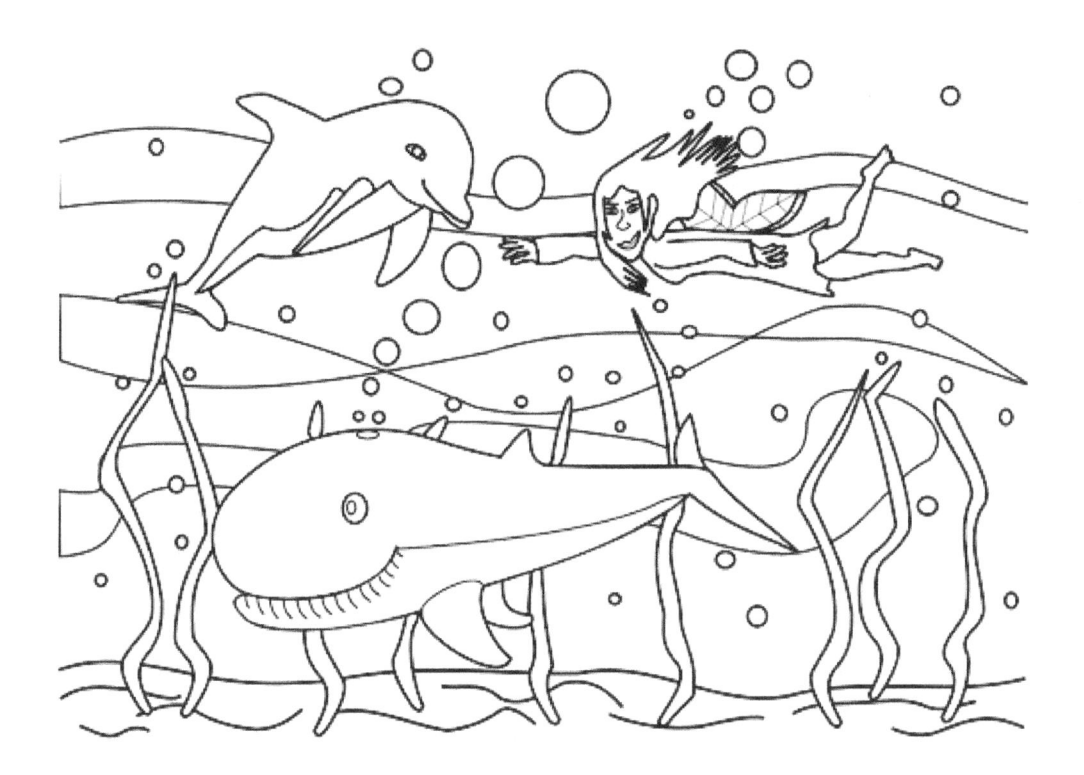

I Can Learn

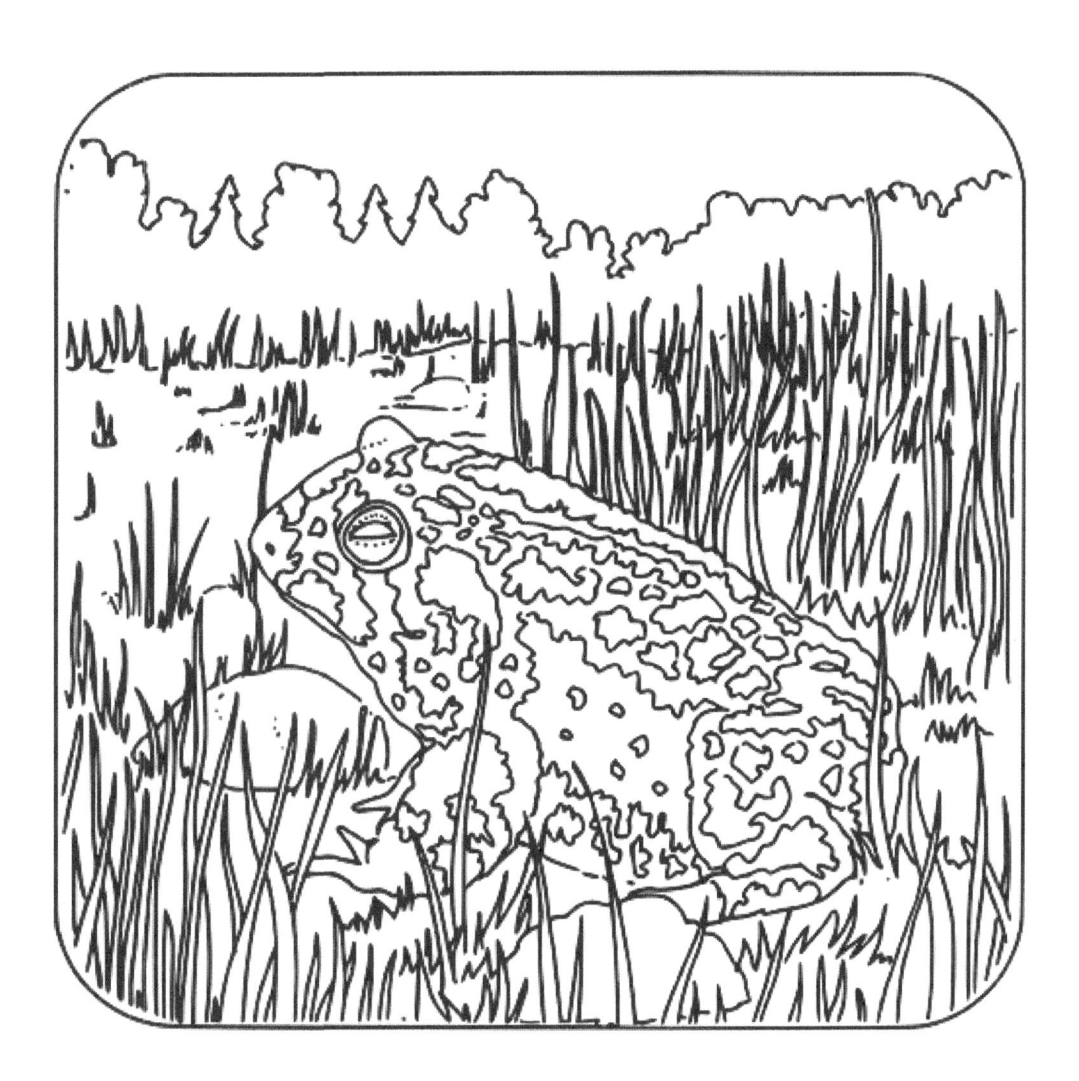

I Tried

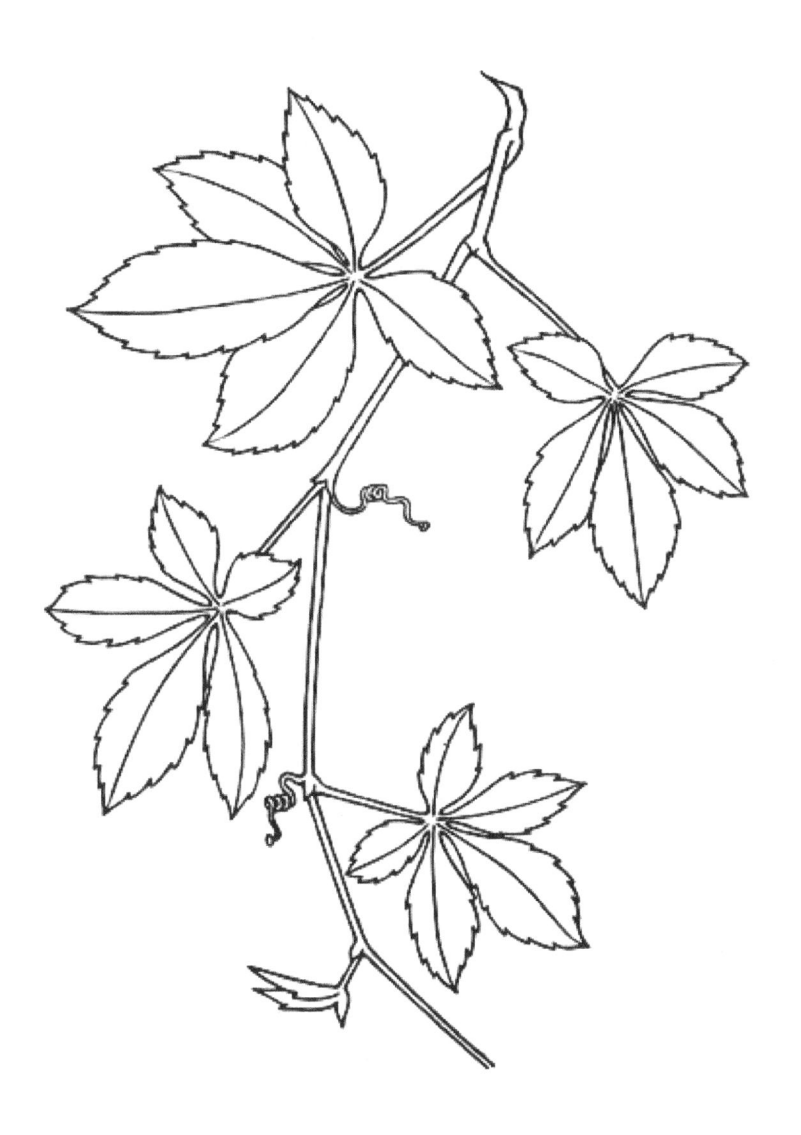

I am Better Now

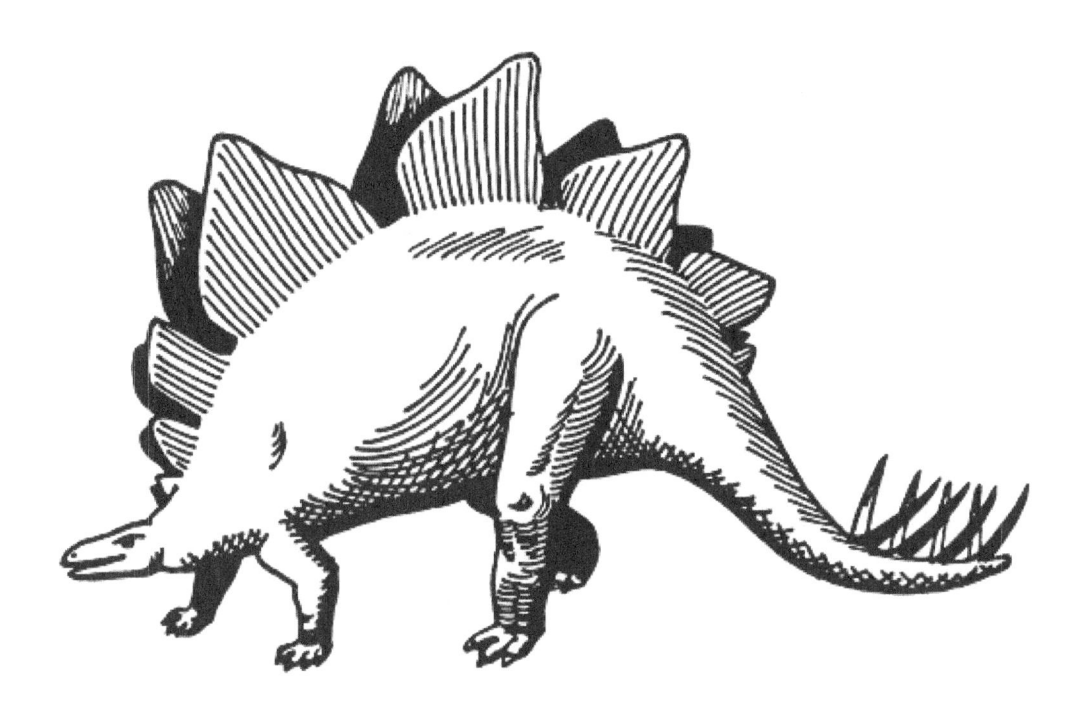

I Can Change

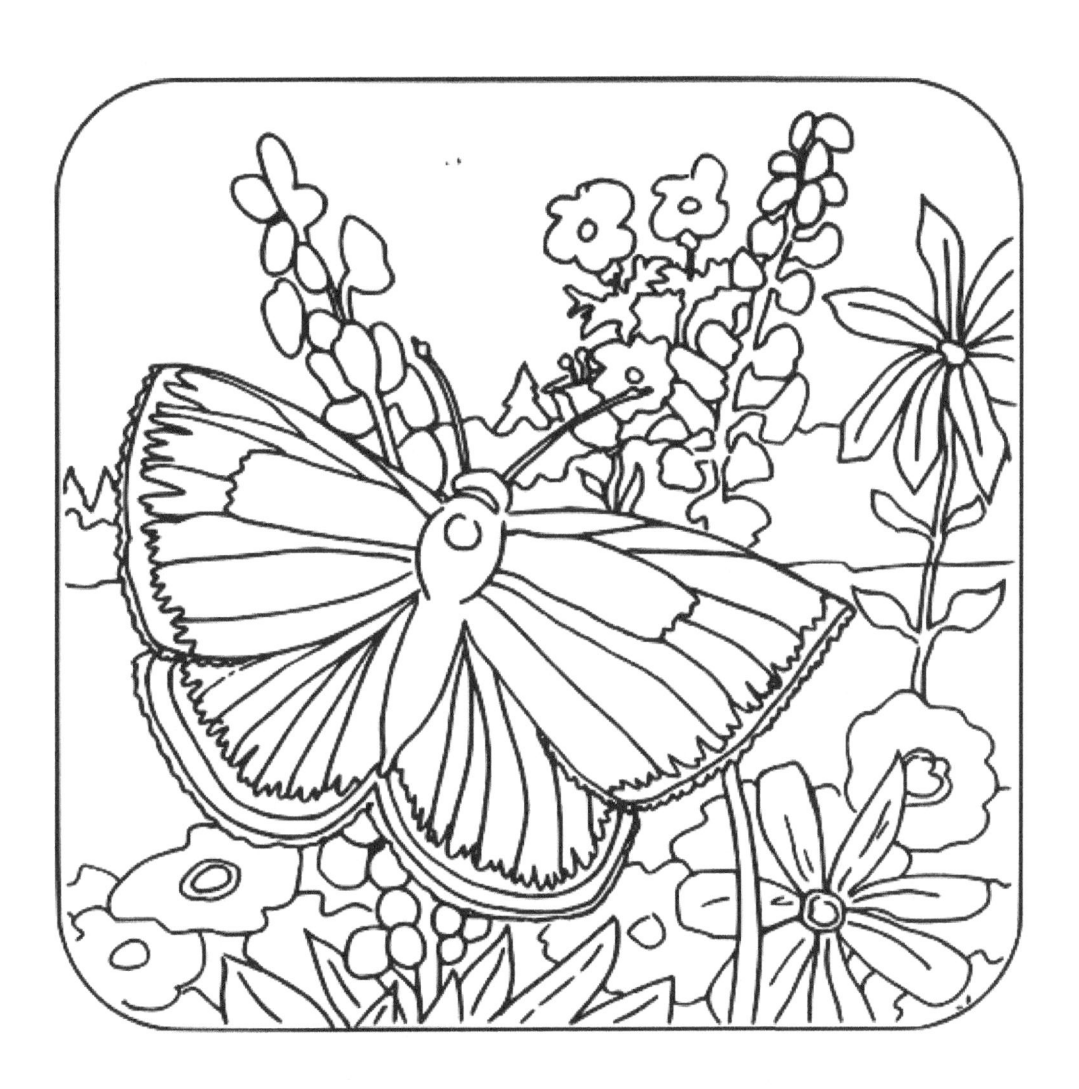

I Deserve Good Things

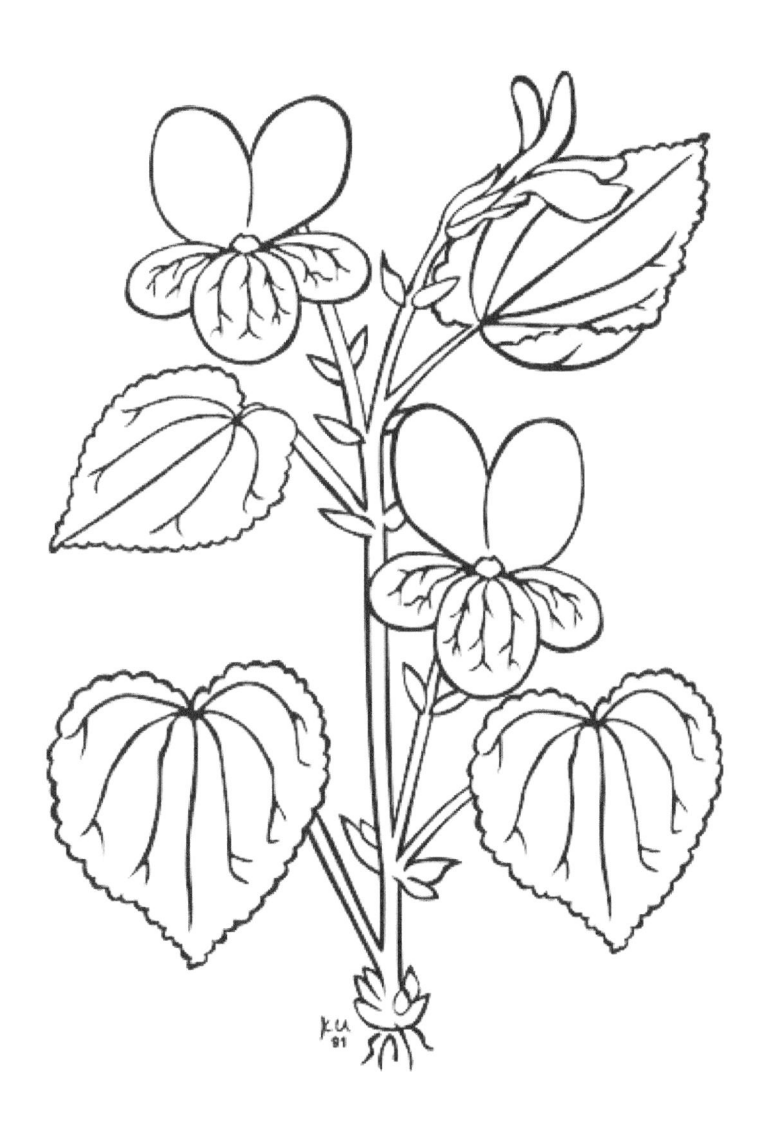

I am Strong Now

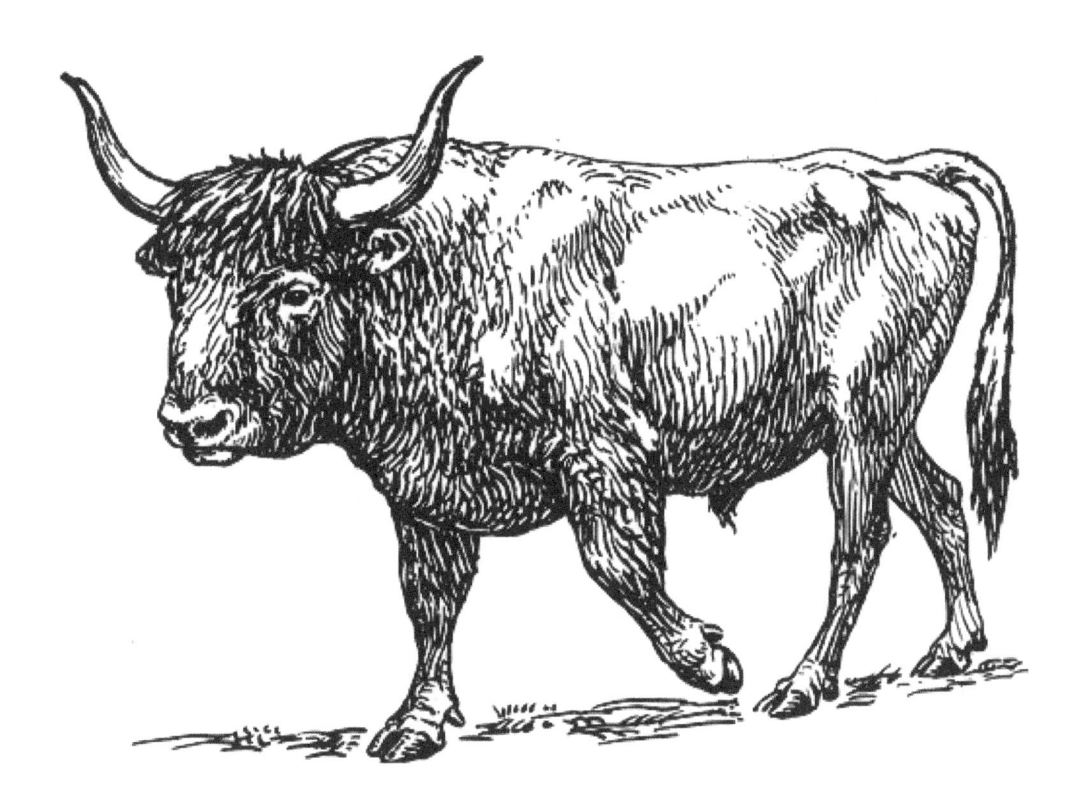

I am Worthy

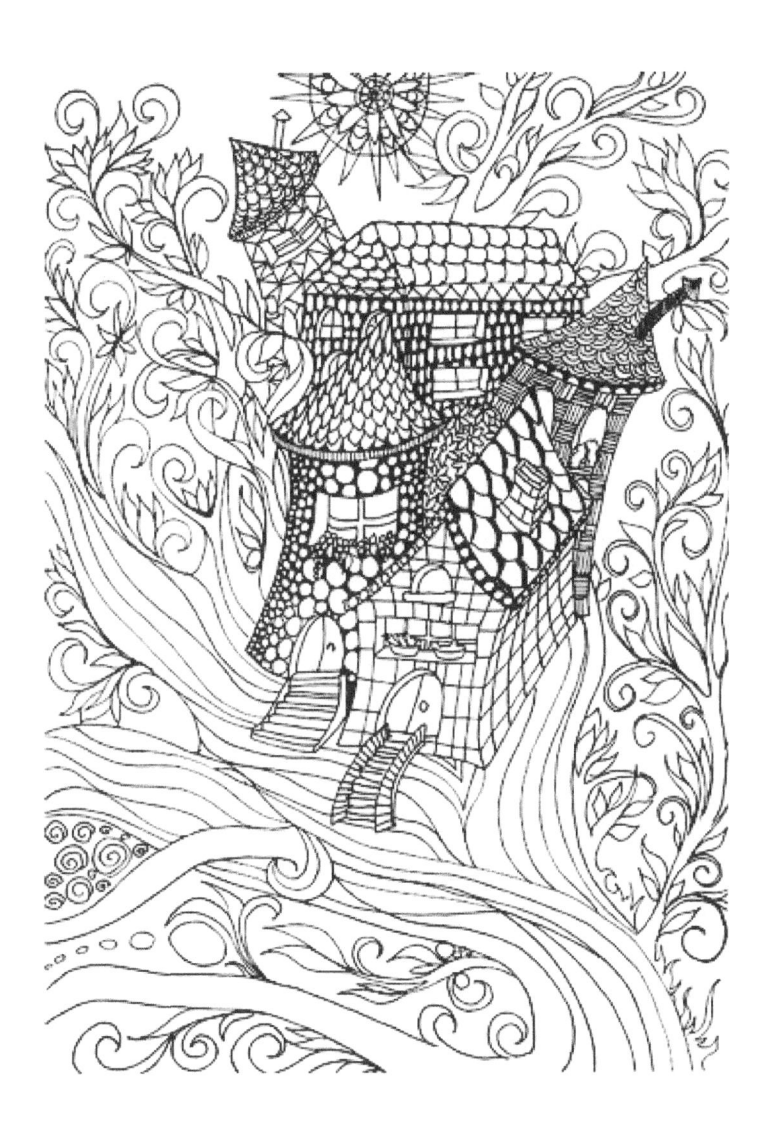

I am Unique

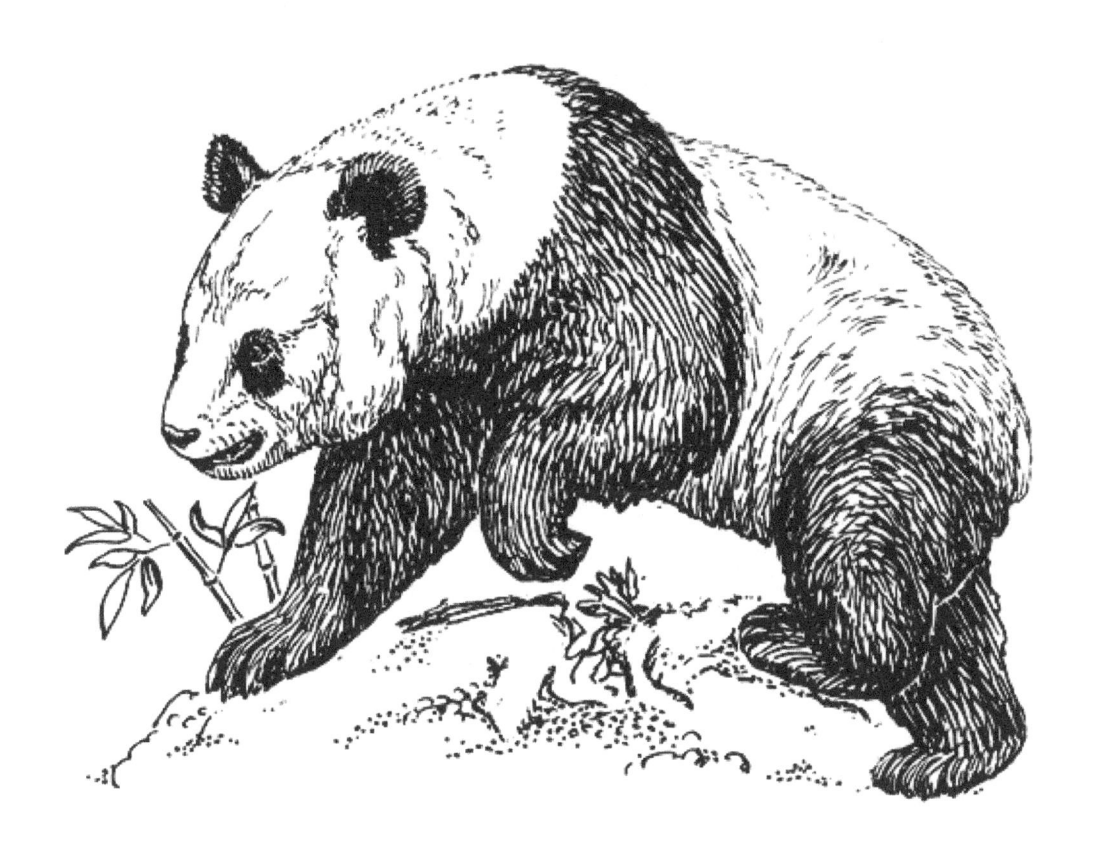

I Can Face my Fears

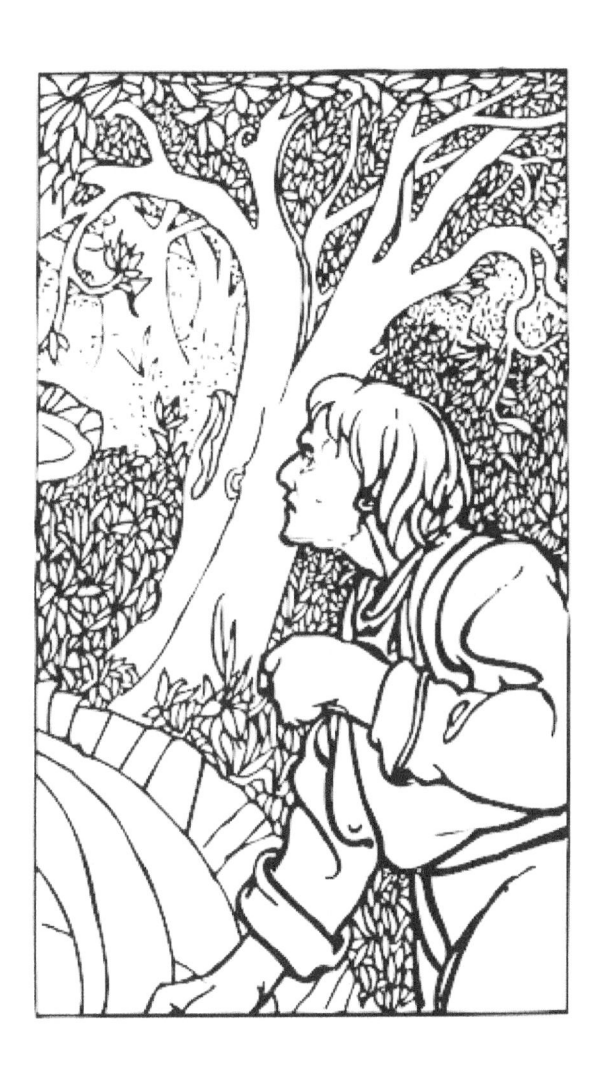

I am Wonderful

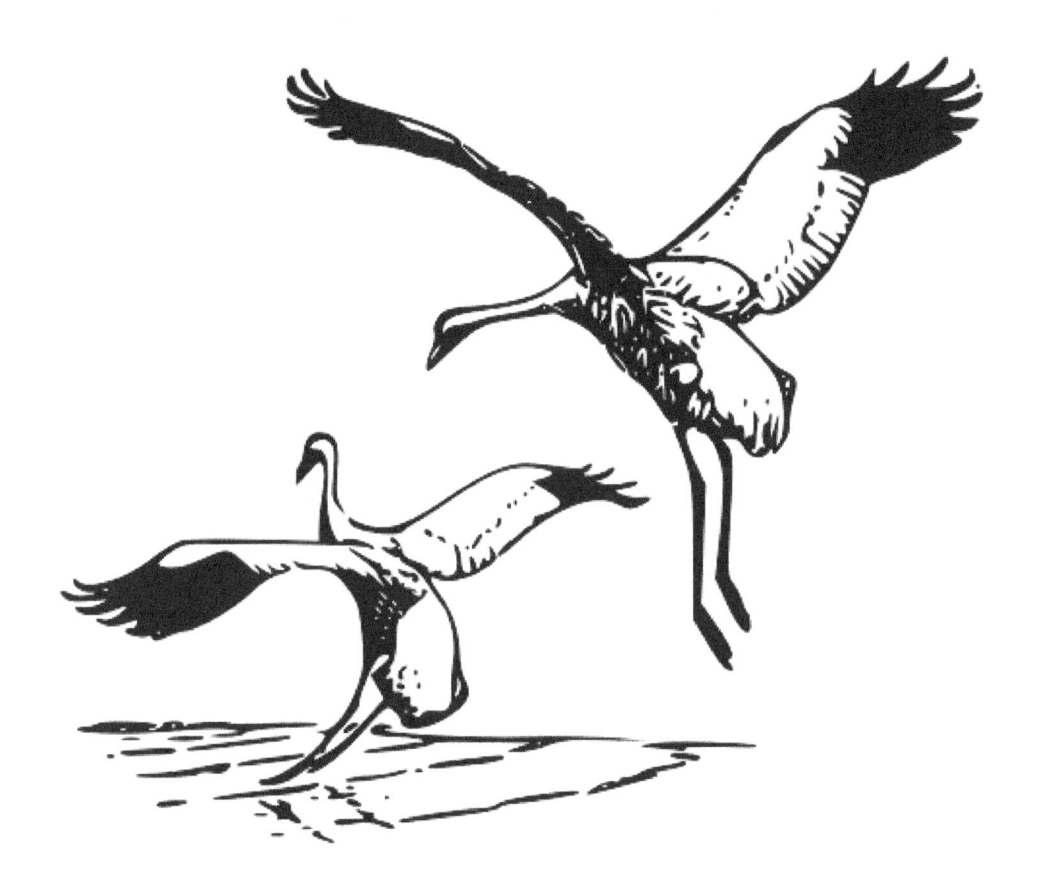

I Can do It

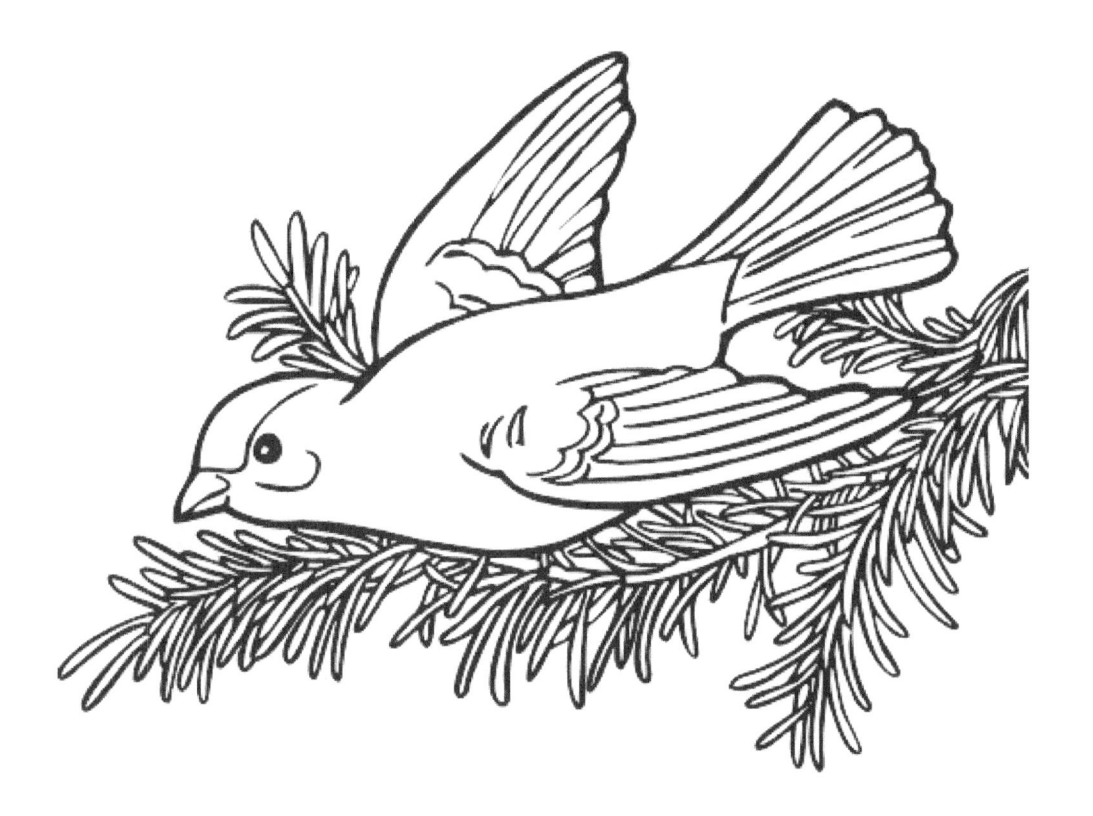

I am Alright

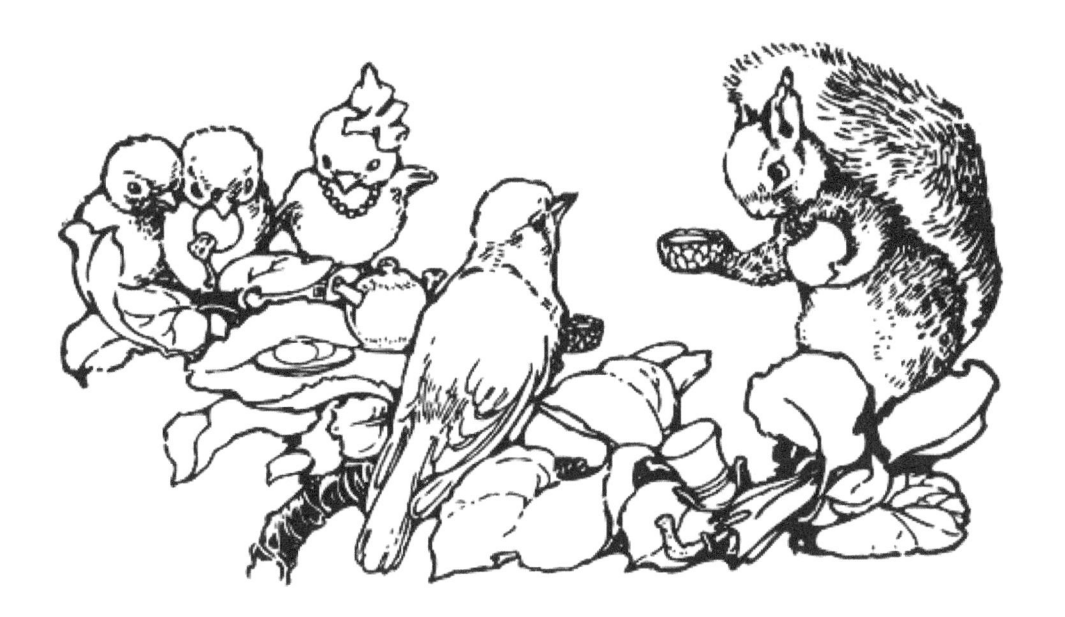

I Believe in Myself

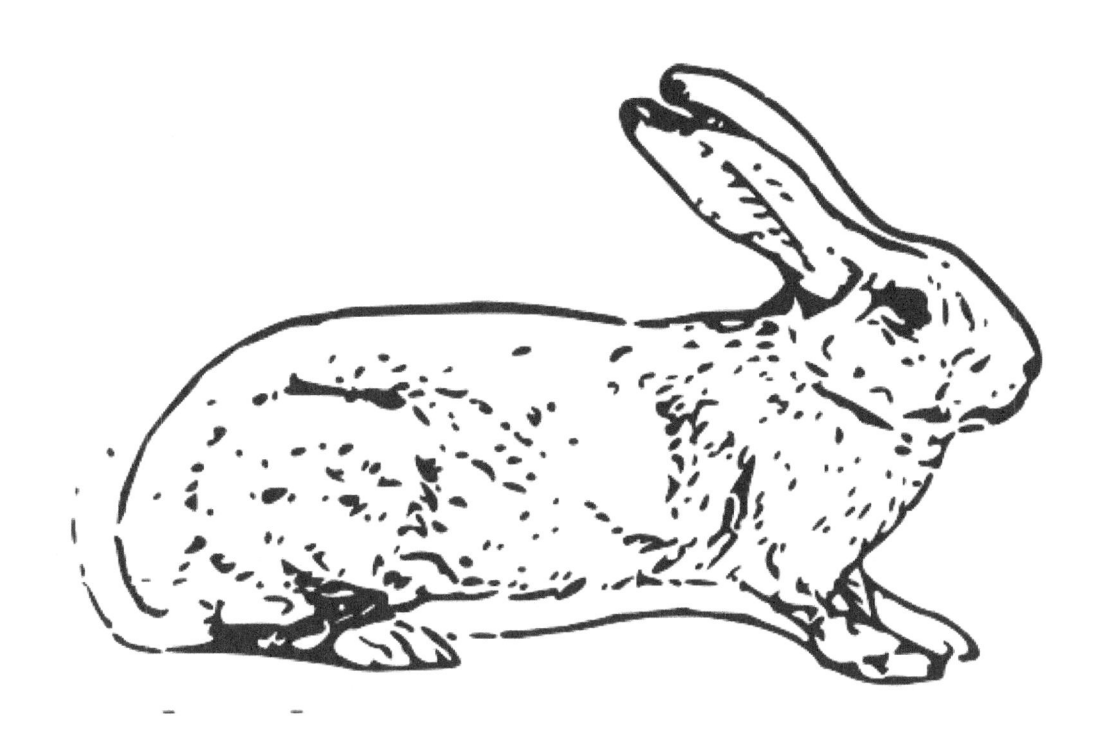

I Can Grow

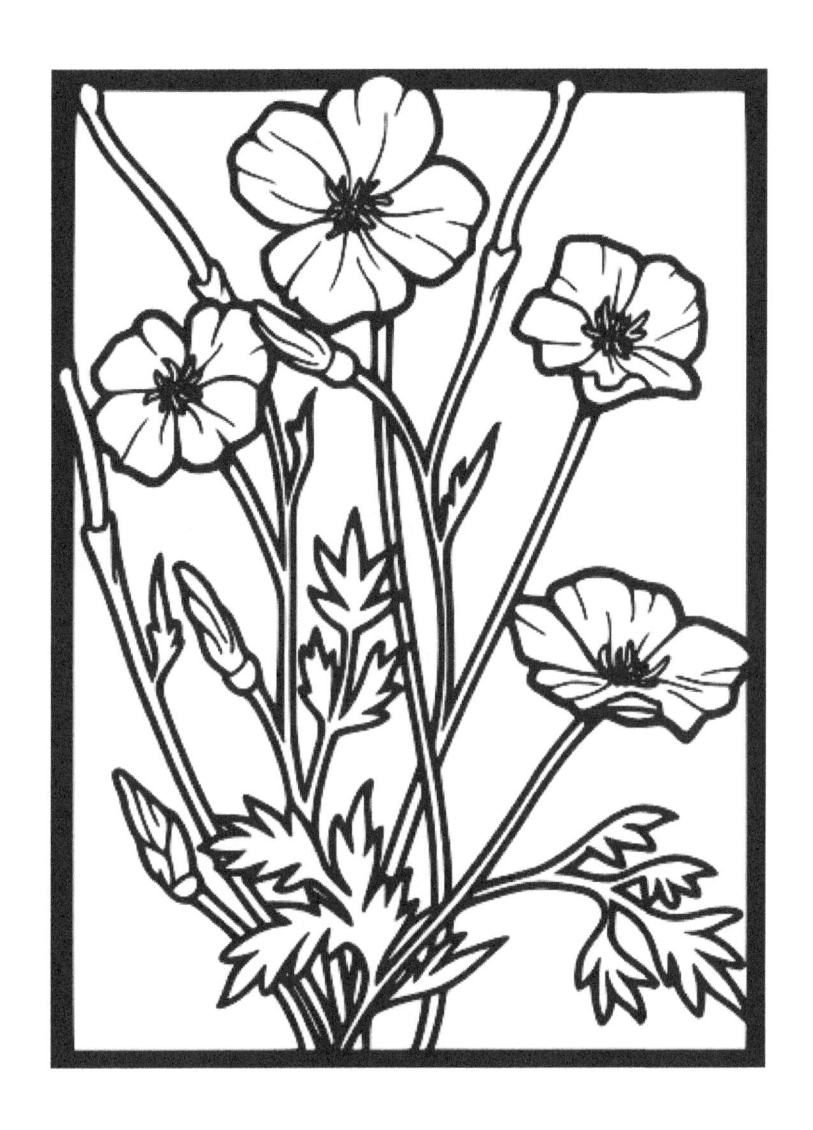

I Can Become Stronger

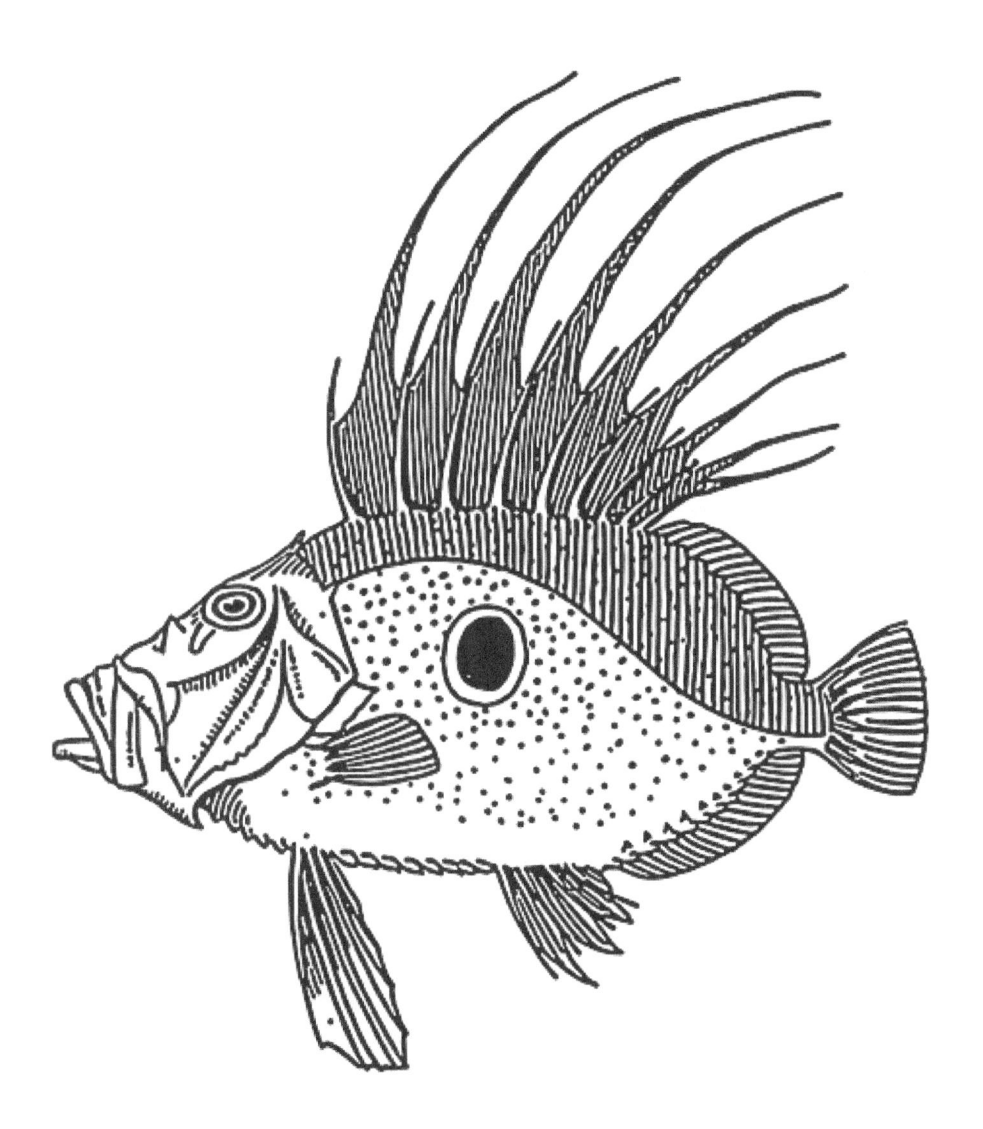

EDITOR BIO

Mark Odland graduated from Augustana College in Sioux Falls, SD, with a B.A. in art and religion. Here he studied drawing, painting, and printmaking under nationally-renowned printmaker Carl Grupp. He went on to earn his M.Div. degree from Luther Seminary in Saint Paul, MN, and his M.A. in Marriage and Family Therapy from the Minnesota School of Professional Psychology in Eagan, MN. An award-winning artist, Mark feels privileged to have his work displayed in various collections around the world. In his work as an EMDR therapist, consultant, and educator, he continues to explore the dynamic intersection between creativity and healing.

CONSULTATION

Mark Odland is able to provide approved EMDR consultation for those desiring to:

1) Become EMDRIA Certified
2) Complete EMDR Basic Training
3) Become an Approved Consultant
4) Discuss Difficult Cases

Mark's education, experience, and ongoing training allow him to provide guidance on a variety of issues during consultation sessions. However, he specializes on the following within EMDR therapy: general practice, spirituality, creativity, childhood abuse and neglect, addiction, and military veterans.

CONTINUING EDUCATION

Mark Odland's continuing education courses are often available as webinars, books, e-books, and audio books. Available to therapists worldwide, his growing list of learning opportunities includes the following subjects:

1) EMDR and Visual Art
2) EMDR and Spiritual Trauma
3) Spiritual Interweaves
4) Spiritual Resource-Building
5) How to Start a Trauma-Focused Private Practice
6) EMDR and Natural Medicine

SPREAD THE WORD

If you enjoyed this book, Mark would be grateful if you left an online review at amazon.com

PURCHASING BOOKS FOR CLIENTS

If you're an EMDR therapist and would like to purchase more copies for clients, you may qualify to receive a discount for bulk purchases. To find out more, send an email to: mark@bilateralinnovations.

PURPOSE

Mark founded Bilateral Innovations with the following purpose:

Bilateral Innovations provides EMDRIA-Approved Consultation and Continuing Education, for the purpose of transforming the world, one client at a time.

To learn more, please visit his website at: bilateralinnovations.com

Made in the USA
Las Vegas, NV
15 January 2024